Dr. Atkins'
Health Manifesto
• • • • • • • • • • • • • • • • •

The One Hidden Cause of Most Modern Illness...
and HOW TO DEFEAT IT!

D1355174

by Robert C. Atkins, M.D.

For additional copies or questions, please contact a Member Services Representative at Dr. Atkins' Health Revelations, P.O. Box 1051, Fort Erie, ON L2A 4N8. You may also call 1(410)783-8440 or send a fax to 1(410)783-8438.

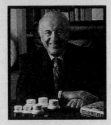

Meet
Dr. Robert C. Atkins

Trained in cardiology at the prestigious Cornell University Medical College, Dr. Robert C. Atkins began his journey away from orthodox medicine toward Complementary Medicine in 1963, after he personally experienced the health benefits accompanying his weight loss on a low-carbohydrate diet. This diet has become the most effective weight-loss program of the 20th Century. His quest for nutritionally-based treatments led to the inescapable truth: working with nature is better than opposing it.

Since then, he has become a world leader in effective nutrition-based treatments for cancer, heart disease, hypoglycemia, diabetes, arthritis, cholesterol, chronic fatigue, asthma, colitis, obesity, and more. He has adopted hundreds of alternative healing methods, including herbal medicine, acupuncture, homeopathy, chelation therapy, bioenergetics and a variety of healing arts that are all safer than those in common medical use.

Dr. Atkins' practice has grown from a busy one-man operation to a large medical center in the heart of New York City. He is now North America's leading practitioner of Complementary Medicine, with 60,000 patients spanning a career of 30-plus years. His practice embraces every valid healing art, including valid naturopathy, chiropractic, oriental medicine and neurolinguistics, along with physicians trained in most medical specialties.

The internationally renowned Atkins Center for Complementary Medicine draws on a wide range of techniques that complement each other and increase the patient's probability of successful healing. Orthodox medicine is not rejected. Rather, it is enhanced by these safe, effective methods.

In addition to his practice, Dr. Atkins is the host of WOR's *Design for Living*, North America's longest-running radio health program, and the host of the nationally syndicated radio show *Your Health Choices*.

Former President of the Foundation for the Advancement of Innovative Medicine, Dr. Atkins is the author of *Dr. Atkins' New Diet Revolution* (currently on the New York Times Best Sellers List), *Dr. Atkins' Diet Revolution*, and *Dr. Atkins' Health Revolution* and the recipient of numerous awards. He is a winner of Pioneer Awards from the National Health Federation and the Foundation for the Advancement of Innovative Medicine and recipient of the Man of the Year Award from the World Organization of Alternative Medicine.

Dr. Atkins is a true veteran who has worked both sides of the medical fence and saw his patient success rate jump from 25% to 80% when he switched to Complementary Medicine in the 1970s.

Contents

The greatest health problem of our time

....and a breakthrough!

For most of mankind's history, the chief health problems were tiny bugs—parasites and micro-organisms—that caused plague, pneumonia, tuberculosis, malaria, syphilis and other infectious diseases.

But in our century, the entire health picture changed dramatically. Better public sanitation, combined with drugs that attacked and killed the bugs, gave us a decisive edge in the battle against these little micro-organisms. .

By the 1950s, most infectious diseases—the big killers for thousands of years—had been brought under control. Some almost disappeared completely. That was the good news. The bad news was that in the decades to follow doctors began seeing more and more cases of cancer, heart disease, diabetes and other ailments that had been very rare previously. Now we realize that these diseases—including candida, arthritis, headaches, heart rhythm disturbances, multiple sclerosis, irritable bowel, and many others—have reached epidemic proportions.

Almost every single Canadian family has

been affected by one or more of these diseases. They are referred to as "lifestyle diseases," because they are related to where people live, what they do, and what they eat. But no one knows exactly what the relationship is. (People in undeveloped nations generally don't get these diseases at all!)

What's worse, mainstream medicine, with its attack-and-destroy, bug-hunting mentality (that worked so well in the first part of this century) seems totally unsuited to the war against these modern ailments. Despite many billions of dollars spent, there has been almost no progress in bringing them under control.

But within the last 15 years, we have made a major breakthrough. Working with an informal network of clinics, researchers, and individual practitioners all over the world, we have discovered what we believe to be the cause of most of these new ailments. And we have already found dozens of ways to defeat them. Even in cases that are too advanced to cure, we have made great strides in being able to stop them from progressing. Patients who previously were given a death sentence found they could stabilize their illnesses, build up their underlying health, and go on to live happy, productive lives.

You'll read some of their case histories in this booklet, and about the breakthrough that makes them possible.

And you'll also find possible solutions to the major health problems you face.

Please read on....

Dr. Atkins' Health Manifesto:

New hope for victims of cancer, heart disease, diabetes, arthritis, multiple sclerosis, irritable bowel syndrome, hypertension, heart rhythm disturbances, obesity . . . and many more . . .

Most Modern Illness has a Single, Hidden Cause

Here's how to strike at the cause of these illnesses, not just the symptoms . . .

Chapter 1

My Personal Health Revelation

Like any pioneer in a new field, my success did not come easy. I had to learn the hard way.

At 33, I looked 45. I weighed 193 and had three chins. I decided to go on a diet. But of course most diets don't work in the long run, like most other people, I was soon disappointed. So, I did a huge amount of research and found one diet that was different from all of the rest.

It was a simple, no-hunger, eat-all-you-want diet discovered during World War II by the late Dr. Alfred W. Pennington. It zeroed in on two culprits: sugar and starch.

With hopes of losing three pounds in the first six months, I was flabbergasted when I dropped 30! And rather than leaving me weak, it took away most of my lethargy, depression, and fatigue! Spurred on by my own experiences, I then wrote a diet book that sold 10 million copies.

Soon after, yet another event changed my life. I was asked to give a lecture by a group of doctors I had criticized for their deviation from the mainstream. They liked my speech, and they befriended me. One of them asked if I knew cancer treatments were being suppressed. And had I really investigated alternative medicine? I couldn't say I had, and putting aside the arrogant close-mindedness bred into me by my medical education, I began studying chelation therapy, herbal medicine, acupuncture, homeopathy, musculoskeletal techniques, and other neglected branches of medicine.

Not every branch turned out to have fruit on it, of course. Some of them were just downright quackery with little evidence to support them. But after a few years of furious research, I gradually began to see that at least a dozen fields of innovative medicine were producing dynamite results for the few brave, scattered doctors who were using them at that time.

When my new techniques pushed me into the public spotlight, I expanded my practice from a one-man show to a large medical center staffed by skilled healers in naturopathy, chiropractic, oriental medicine, neurolinguistics, immunology, nutritional biochemistry, and most other medical specialties—without ever abandoning my traditional medical training and experience.

The rest, as they say, is history.

Chapter 2

A Major Victory Against Cancer

Let me first introduce you to one of my patients: Denton Brill.*

Denton was a vigorous, active, 52-year-old when he was diagnosed with colon cancer—second only to lung cancer as a major cause of cancer deaths among North American males.

Every year, over 100,000 people get this diagnosis and about 50,000 die within 5 years

After a colonoscopy, Denton was told that he was a "grower." His surgeon had discovered four large polyps. Denton was told that the only treatment for his cancer was chemotherapy—with its devastating side effects.

While chemotherapy may extend the patients life—I guarantee you that those who are subjected to chemotherapy suffer a much sicker and more miserable life.

Fortunately, Denton had done some of his

---

* *I changed all the names in this booklet to protect my patients' privacy.*

own research on the subject. He was not eager to be blasted with chemical agents with a myriad of debilitating side effects. He said a resounding "NO" to this "only" option and looked into complementary medicine.

He was frightened but determined

Denton asked me about the work of Emanuel Revici, of Lawrence Burton, and of Stanislas Burszynski, who have all made splendid contributions to treating cancer.

"That's only the beginning," I told him. *"There's plenty of reason for optimism."* There are a dozen or so other biologic treatments that have to be included. My German colleague, Professor Friedrich Douwes reported over a dozen cures with his biologic therapy, and enzymologist Karl Ransberger had reported on 38 cases of total remission using his world-renowned Wobe-Mugos enzyme.

Denton had a choice after all!

I could see the relief in Denton's face and knew then that he would be a curable *person*. Denton had the two most valuable traits of all— fighting spirit and the emotional unwillingness to accept the idea of being sick.

Kitchen sink complementarism

My plan for treating Denton was the opposite of orthodox medicine. I aimed to build up the body, not tear down the cancer. I planned to use what I call *"kitchen sink complementarism."* In other words, I'd use everything but the kitchen sink to boost his health, stimulate his immune system, and enable his body to heal itself.

I had created a method of treatment that broke away from the orthodox blinders and combined all of the bona fide, clinically tested, effective, and health-enhancing therapies I knew of—including those ignored, dismissed, and suppressed by the establishment. As long as it doesn't hurt, why not try it? The worst that can happen is that some treatments offer nothing that helps. On the other hand, I give the body plenty to choose from. The best thing that can happen is that . . . .

Your body finds what it needs to achieve its own goal of healing

Fortunately, Denton's immune system was intact—he had not let his oncologist subject him to the debilitating effects of chemotherapy.

The first step was to get him on a health-enhancing diet. I prescribed a diet that cut back on carbohydrates and eliminated sugar and chemical additives.

The second course of action included individualized enzyme and antioxidant therapy. This included supplementing with an array of effective vitamins, minerals, and herbs. He also received alternating treatments of our mistletoe formula with dosages of 714X and Ukraine.

Slowly, after many ups and downs, Denton made real progress! Within a year of my kitchen sink therapy...

. . . Denton proudly proclaimed, *"I feel better than ever!"*

CT scans came out completely negative! And when he went for another colonoscopy—no signs of malignancy were found!

Today, 3 years after he first came to see me, Denton lives *more* than a normal life—holding down two jobs. *"I know there is no more cancer,"* Denton says. *"And I'm looking forward to 60 more years of life—and then some!"*

That's not all...

Denton succeeded before coming close to the bottom of my sink. There's much, much more...*Iscador / Helixor, Carnivora, DC4, ozone, Koch's glyoxylide, thymosin, Hoxsey's herbs, pancreatic enzymes, shark cartilage,* and dozens more.

And don't forget the aforementioned treatments of Dr. Burton, Dr. Revici, Dr. Burszynski, nor William Donald Kelley and Andrew Ivy, nor the countless others who have been forgotten and suppressed by the cancer establishment.

Unproven does *not* mean disproven!

Most treatments that become victims of the cancer establishment get placed on the American Cancer Society's "unproven methods" list, otherwise known as "cancer quackery." To the American Cancer Society, unproven is disproven.

I, on the other hand, view unproven as an opportunity. I choose to scour the lists for promising yet-to-be-proven therapies and jump at the opportunity to consider their possible benefits in helping to treat my patients.

Denton Brill's success was achieved with the help of unproven therapies. If he had been intimidated by the establishment, and opted for proven only, he would have gone through months, even years, of debilitating side effects from a treatment far from being guaranteed to work.

Chapter 3

A Diet for Much More than Weight Loss

Most people know me as the creator of the Atkins Diet. I owe most of my fame and fortune to my first book *Dr. Atkins' Diet Revolution*. As one of only two diet books listed on the Top 50 All Time Mass Market Best Sellers, *Diet Revolution* was translated into every major language and read by millions of people all over the world—more than 10 million copies were sold.

That was over twenty years ago. Since then, I have dedicated my life's work to using nutrition to treat serious health problems. My diet has become a crucial part of my healing program. You can't be healthy if you don't eat right, and if you do eat right, you should be able to maintain a healthy weight.

I, too, was a victim of the low-fat food fraud

I came upon my diet when I realized that I had a weight problem. I wanted to lose some pounds. So like anyone else, I did the logical things. I started on a typical low-fat, low-calorie diet.

But I didn't like it. Because I was tired and hungry all of the time!

That experience led me to a quarter of a century of research and clinical and personal trials into an area where most doctors fear to tread—for reasons I will explain.

At first, I was just trying to understand why some people gained weight and others didn't. I was trying to find an easy, painless way for those of us who have a tendency to add pounds, to lose weight and keep it off.

I looked for a system, an approach that was as close to nature as possible. Animals in the wild do not become obese. Surely there was a more natural diet that would do the same thing for humans.

The first—and only effective— *all-you-can-eat* diet

I soon found it. A diet that lets people eat pretty much all they want—and still lose weight. Not only can you eat as much as you want...you can also eat a lot of the food that is forbidden on other diet plans.

Eggs, for example, eat all you want.

Meat, yes, red meat...and chicken, and ham...you can eat all you want.

And butter! Throw out the margarine. This diet lets you eat butter. And guess what? It can also reduce your blood pressure and your likelihood of having heart trouble...

And calories in general. This diet lets many people give up calorie counting...and yet, still lose weight.

Yes, I was just looking for a way to lose weight. And this diet did the trick (I'll tell you more in a moment) but I suspected it did more than that.

You are what you eat

I had a hunch that getting your eating habits in tune with a more natural diet might produce some other benefits. Diet surely had an impact on what we call "lifestyle" or modern illnesses. It was so obvious. A "lifestyle" ailment would have to be addressed with a lifestyle solution-like diet. But no one, to my knowledge, had ever thoroughly researched the issue. They barely teach nutrition at all in medical school. And, in general, the medical establishment is dead set against nutritional or dietary remedies. (More about that in a moment, too.)

What amazed and delighted me was that I discovered that my weight-loss diet did far more than just help people lose pounds.

A gateway into a world of nutritional medicine

My diet proved to be the foundation for an entirely new healing approach—one which brought results better than practically anyone else was getting. I'm not talking about infectious disease...though it does help make people generally more healthy and better able to fight all sorts of disease.

Where my diet really showed its merit was against the very intractable...often incurable...modern illnesses—such as diabetes, cancer, heart disease, arthritis, irritable bowel syndrome, multiple sclerosis, hypertension, PMS, headaches, candida, and hypoglycemia.

Let me tell you just a few of the results we have had:

Diabetes—8 out of 10 of the people who come to the Atkins Center with Type II diabetes are able to throw away their dangerous diabetes drugs, such as Drabanese, Micronase and Glucotrol, within 8 weeks.

Unstable heart arrhythmias—Over half of the people who come in to the Atkins Center with an unstable heart arrhythmia are able to throw away their killer beta blockers within 4 weeks.

Heart disease—We have demonstrated reversal of the symptoms of heart disease in over 85% of Atkins Center overweight coronary patients who have diligently followed our program consistently.

Hypertension—Our success in freeing people of the burden of unnecessary and deadly blood pressure drugs is at least over 80%.

Irritable bowel syndrome—Our treatment regimen has yielded an 80% improvement rate in a population made up primarily of treatment failures of other physicians. Our patients are happy to toss their dangerous steroid drugs in the garbage within a few weeks.

Why should you listen to me?

Over 60,000 patients have come through my clinic in New York since we opened the doors in 1970. I'll match our healing results against the best in the world.

I'm not saying this to brag. I just want to point out that there is a reason for this that has nothing to do with me personally. I try to do my best with every patient. But so do most doctors.

My success comes from an insight that we developed many years ago...one which has proven itself over and over again.

You see, as we watched more and more people come through the clinic and leave with their health problems resolved, or at least in better shape than they went in, we began experimenting. We didn't stray from the basic nutritional principles that I laid out in my 1972 book because they have proven themselves to work.

We keep moving ahead

We added things. Because other doctors were experimenting too, all over the world. They were trying natural, safe substances...often with impressive results.

We kept our eyes and ears open so we could bring patients the work of 100s of cutting-edge researchers.

We've studied the work of break-through researchers, like Dr. Hans Nieper. He was gracious enough to share with me his discovery of what I view as the first substance therapeutically effective in treating most cases of multiple sclerosis—the key mineral transporter, calcium AEP. Dr. Nieper has successfully treated over 1,500 cases with this calcium salt. Bringing the progressive nature of this disease to a halt.

And the breakthrough research of my German colleague *Professor Friedrich Douwes*. Professor Douwes reported over a dozen cures of pancreatic cancer with his biologic therapy.

Then there are the invaluable contributions of the late nutritional pioneer **Carlton Fredericks, Ph.D.**, who was the acknowledged patriarch of clinical nutrition. He devised the first *nutritional* protocols for over-estrogenized women and for those with low-estrogen conditions, eliminating the need for prescription hormones.

Those are only a few of the natural, safe, effective therapies being used around the world.

We've tried thousands of the alternative healers that show promise

As long as they are completely harmless... my attitude is: "If there's a substance that works, and is completely harmless, then I want to add it to my healing arsenal."

And in many cases, the results are very impressive:

➤ **Antioxidants**, for example, have been proven to help slow down the aging process and to reverse the degenerative diseases of aging, including cancer, cardiovascular disease, Alzheimer's disease, diabetes, pulmonary disease, and just about everything else.

➤ **Gamma-linolenic acid (GLA) nutrients** (especially primrose oil)—One of the most brilliant minds in Complementary Medicine Dr. David Horrobin has proved via double-blind, controlled studies that GLA is the most effective treatment yet for PMS, atopic eczema in children, the dry eye syndrome, and Sjogren's syndrome. These studies virtually prove its value in many allergy and immune disorders, in lowering hypertension and cholesterol, in aiding alcoholism, in breast tenderness, in Raynaud's syndrome, in diabetic neuropathy, in rheumatoid arthritis and in autoimmune disorders such as MS, lupus, and scleroderma. It has also been tested and shown to have favorable results in hyperactive children, depression, schizophrenia, and Parkinsonism. Animal studies have shown a possible benefit in treating cancer.

➤ **Omega-3 fatty acids (DHA, EPA)**— Studies have proven that EPA, in large enough doses, has the power to single-handedly wipe out the lucrative antihypertensive market and the anticholesterol market. I've found it invaluable in treating cancer, arthritis, allergy, MS, and more. It is particularly valuable in lowering elevated triglyceride levels.

➤ **Mineral Transporters (orotates, aspartates, and EAP)** are invaluable in optimizing the body's absorption of much-needed minerals, such as magnesium. As a cardiologist, I am unrestrainedly enthusiastic over magnesium orotate in just about any cardiovascular condition imaginable. Calcium-EAP should be used to replace the most dangerous drugs in the entire medical profession—immunosuppressive drugs. I've seen it work wonders in treating arthritis. Dr. Nieper has proven its value in treating juvenile diabetes, gastritis and Crohn's disease, erythema nodosum, thyroiditis, myocarditis, or sarcoid.

➤ **Taurine**—This amino acid works exceptionally well in helping to lower high cholesterol levels and high blood pressure. Studies also show that it seems able to help control heart rhythm irregularities. Most importantly, taurine has been proven to help in the treatment of epilepsy. At the Atkins Center, we have been able to get at least 40 percent of patients with seizure disorder off their medications.

➤ **Carnitine's** greatest success is in the treatment of coronary insufficiency. It has also been shown to benefit cardiomyopathies and unstable heart rhythms, to decrease serum triglyceride and cholesterol levels, and to increase HDL (*International Journal of Cardiology,* vol. 5, 1984).

➤ **Bromelain**—Over 200 scientific papers have been published showing bromelain's positive effect as a digestive aid, anti-inflammatory agent, and smooth muscle relaxer. It has been used for ulcer prevention, sinusitis relief, as a pain reliever, and more. It's most powerful effect, when used in large enough dosages, is in treating and preventing atherosclerosis.

➤ **Coenzyme Q10** should top the list of any heart treatment program. It has been proven to help in treating cardiovascular disease, hypertension, high blood pressure, angina, diabetes mellitus, heart rhythm disturbances, and cardiomyopathy. It's amazing that orthodox medicine doesn't give it the time of day—how could they possibly ignore the list of proven benefits? (*The Miracle Nutrient Coenzyme Q10,* Bantum Books, 1986).

➤ **Quercetin** is perhaps the most effective antioxidant for fighting the effects of chemical sensitivity, often characterized by a persistent headache. It has been shown to benefit hypertension and to reduce small strokes. It is also one of the few nutrients ever shown to help treat varicose veins (*Biochemical Pharmacology*, vol. 33, 1984).

➤ **Pantethine**—Besides it's success in treating candidiasis and alcoholism, pantethine plays a pivotal role in cholesterol metabolism. It has also been proven to help treat heart disease and to suppress platelet clumping (*Current Therapeutic Research*, vol. 38, 1985).

➤ **Octacosanol**—Research has identified octacosanol as the active ingredient in wheat germ, responsible for improving stamina, reaction time, and cardiovascular responses. It has also been proven to improve brain function, memory deficit, Alzheimer's, Parkinson's, seizure disorder, multiple sclerosis, children's attention deficit disorder, and more (*Annals of Neurology*, vol. 16, 1984).

The list of safe, effective healers gets longer and longer every day. And every day, we find out a little more and where and when these healing agents work best.

Our results keep getting better all the time!

Let me stop right here and get something off my chest.

There's a big difference between healing these modern diseases and healing the diseases of 100 years ago.

Alexander Fleming was able to isolate bacteria in a petri dish and then see what it took to kill it. It was a simple, scientifically-speaking, procedure. You could do the test over and over again...and verify the results.

The drug companies keep trying to do the same thing for modern ailments—and usually fail miserably. When it was noticed that high cholesterol levels were associated with heart disease, they began looking for drugs that would keep cholesterol levels down. Isolating a single factor—cholesterol counts—made it possible to produce drugs, prove that they lowered cholesterol counts, and get them approved by the FDA.

The drugs worked! They lowered cholesterol levels. Only, the patients died just the same.

We still don't know if high cholesterol levels cause heart disease. All we know is that people with heart disease tend to have high cholesterol levels, too. And we know that people on cholesterol-lowering drugs generally die at about the same rate as the patients who don't take the drugs.

I'll give you another example of this phenomenon. A lot of people have heart rhythm disturbances. Most of the time, these are not serious health concerns. But sometimes, the heart goes into fibrillation and stops doing its job altogether.

So, once again, the drug companies isolated the problem and went to work. They came up with a drug that did just what they wanted. It stopped the irregularities in the heartbeat. It proved it could do this, and was given FDA approval, and was subsequently widely prescribed for people with this complaint.

Once again, in the real world, with real patients, a problem arose

People who were taking this drug began dying at a much higher rate than before. Their heart beats were regular. But they dropped dead. And the drug was quietly removed from the market.

My point is this:

The real test of any medical procedure or drug is whether or not it helps individual people get better. Unfortunately, you often can't isolate the health problem, or the treatment.

If a patient lacks faith in the doctor, even a good treatment may fail. On the other hand, a good doctor can often get good results from even a bad treatment.

Also, with these modern ailments, we are dealing with delicate internal balances that are affected by almost everything...principally by what you eat, but also by your body's natural metabolism, by your weight, by your eating and exercise habits, by your social life, and so on and so forth. Each patient, and each situation, is different. You can't do a neat little double-blind test, in other words.

But neither can you ignore the fact that people are getting better!

Our patients were getting better in droves...but why?

At first, we didn't know why. We were treating them as individuals, which made it hard to generalize. But we began to put together the pieces of the greatest health puzzle of our time—what causes the huge increase in modern disease: heart complications, diabetes, candidiasis, cancer, multiple sclerosis, IBS, arthritis, stroke, obesity, chronic fatigue, Crohn's disease/colitis, Meniere's disease, gall bladder disease, infertility, peptic ulcer, and more.

We have had many, many patients come to us with these problems—thousands of them. After all, they're the most common major health challenges of our era.

And we've seen dramatic improvement. In many cases, recoveries almost as miraculous as the one I began this booklet telling you about.

But, perhaps more importantly, we noticed a common thread running through these major diseases—a thread that connected the diseases one to another...and showed why our original insight behind the Atkins' diet worked to cure and control these modern illnesses.

Chapter 4

The Hidden Cause Behind Most Modern Disease

There is an entirely new academic discipline emerging. It's called Darwinian Medicine. The idea is to apply the lessons of Darwin's Theory of Evolution to the problems of modern medicine.

One of the things that Darwinian researchers do is to ask themselves what were the conditions under which mankind evolved...and how are they different now? The answers to these questions often produce some striking insights.

But I won't dwell on these. I just want to point out that over many millions of years, God and Nature perfected an animal—we humans—that was well adapted to its environment.

I can't emphasize strongly enough that nature really did provide for us very well. Even before the onset of agriculture, the human animal was able, for millions of years, to remain strong and healthy in conditions of often savage deprivation by eating the fish and animals that scampered and swam around him, and the fruits and vegetables and berries that grew nearby. Without medicine, without expertise, without insulated housing or reliable heating, we nevertheless survived.

> **" The average Canadian consumes about 120 lbs. of sugar each year!"**

We were immensely aided by the fact that the dietary side of our primitive lifestyle was enormously healthy.

How was that diet remarkably different from what we eat today?

In many ways, our diets are better than they ever were. We have more and better foods to choose from—including far more access to refined carbohydrates.

The first sugar refineries in Europe weren't built until Napoleon's time. It was he who had them put up. Until that time, at the beginning of the 19th century...the average European consumed only about 7 pounds of sugar every year. At first, sugar was very expensive and difficult to obtain. But, by the end of the 19th century, the industrial revolution and railroad transportation brought affordable sugar to nearly everyone. Today, the average Canadian consumes about 120 pounds. Or 17 times as much.

This explosion of sugar usage directly corresponds to the explosion in the number of modern ailments reported. Heart disease, diabetes, cancer—these things barely appeared in the medical literature until the 20th century, and then they took off.

What's the connection?

Good question.

Feeding the insulin lion

You could think of your body as a furnace. It's a primitive way to look at it...but it does the job.

When you sit down to a meal, you load the furnace with fuel. This produces the power you need to live. Sugar is loaded with calories— a measure of the heat it will produce. Notice the energy you feel after eating a lot of sugar. A little later you have a letdown feeling...as the sugar levels in your bloodstream fall. You may feel tired, or even subdued or cranky before the next meal.

This power surge you feel after a lot of sugar is a little unnatural. We humans weren't designed for such high-octane fuel. Over the millions of years of our evolution, we ate meat and fresh fruits, vegetables, nuts and berries. It wasn't until fairly recent times that grains made up a large part of our diets...much less refined carbohydrates and sugars!

The glucose rollercoaster ride

So, our cave-man bodies had big jobs to do in adapting to 20th century diets—and, in particular, to high doses of sugar.

When we eat sugar, our bodies get a flare up of energy...with high sugar levels in our blood. But in order to regulate this sugar intake, we produce insulin to bring the sugar level back down to where it is supposed to be.

Most people have a totally incorrect view of the most common form of diabetes, adult-onset diabetes, for example, when they think the body doesn't produce enough insulin. Actually, it produces too much, in an effort to control the blood sugar, and eventually gets overwhelmed and worn out.

Think again about putting fuel into an engine or furnace. Now imagine that the octane is 17 times higher than the machine was designed for. It won't take long before something burns up, burns out, or blows up!

This is essentially what happens in patients with diabetes. They go through the energy flare-ups, the mood swings, the fatigue and low spirits over and over again. By the fifth decade of their lives we begin to see the disease which we can diagnose as Type II diabetes. But the actual cause—inappropriate levels of blood sugar—has been with the patient for many years.

And this analysis suggests a simple prescription:

Cut back on the sugar!

At the Atkins Center, that's exactly what we prescribe. Along with a lot of other safe, natural health boosters that improve overall wellbeing and rev-up the immune system. Unfortunately, as you will see, you can't put the toothpaste back in the tube. The patient will never be totally free of the problem.

But it can be contained—without dangerous drugs. Patients don't have to lead lives of invalids. They don't have to worry about losing their toes. They don't have to worry about the life-threatening effects of the prescription drugs, such as Orinase, that most doctors routinely prescribe to suppress the symptoms. They won't have to worry about symptoms at all... because they'll be attacking the problem at the real cause.

Regulating sugar levels isn't just for diabetics

I have been talking about diabetes, but I want you to know that the blood sugar/insulin relationship—regulating the fire in the furnace—is critical to our health. If this relationship is out of balance, especially for a long time, it affects a great many other critical processes in the body.

In short, when you have a fundamental imbalance...a fundamental problem such as blood sugar levels that are too high for your body to cope with...things start to go wrong. Some of them in ways that don't appear connected at first. But upon closer inspection, the connections begin to show up...as you will see.

That is why I have found that I can work wonders—sometimes near-miracles—simply by restoring this fundamental balance in the body...putting the blood sugar/insulin relationship back to where nature intended it to be.

➢ **If you are often tired for no apparent reason....**I believe I can restore your energy levels to what they should be.

➢ **If you have headaches...**I have a simple cure that cuts their frequency in half. Or if you have children with migraine headaches (an increasing problem!) we've managed to eliminate 93% of them just by making dietary changes.

➢ **If you or someone you know suffers from osteoporosis,** you should know that calcium or estrogen supplements probably wont help. But we've found that the mineral magnesium can turn the tide.

➢ **If you suffer from cancer...**don't give up...most of the cancer patients I have treated have discovered they could fight cancer to a draw...stop it...contain it...and go on to live happy carefree lives....

➢ **If you're crippled by the pain of arthritis...**you don't have to live the rest of your life on toxic drugs...despite what the Arthritis Foundation will tell you, diet does help! I can tell you what foods to avoid...and 3 foods that can help eliminate your pain overnight.

➤ **If you experience periods of memory deficit, brain fog, or fear of Alzheimer's disease...**I have a "smart fat" that can put your mind at ease.

➤ **If you are worried about heart attack...**or have an irregular heartbeat, or any kind of heart ailment...you'll be astonished at the results we have to offer...simply by addressing the fundamental imbalance of blood sugar/insulin and building up the body's natural health mechanisms.

Or, if you just want a simple way to control your weight without giving up eating as much good food as you like, I guarantee this will produce quick, impressive results and a lifetime of health benefits. Weight loss was what got me started. And even if it did no more than that, it would still be an important help to millions of people.

But the benefits go far beyond losing weight.

Chapter 5

The Biggest Mistake Most Doctors Make

I believe most doctors have gone completely wrong. They've made a serious mistake that has severely limited their ability to heal their patients, in my opinion—but you judge for yourself.

Almost all medicine practiced in North America today is based on a model developed early in this century—when the most important thing to doctors and patients was defeating infection. If you caught pneumonia or were seriously injured on the farm, your chances of survival were not great. Because doctors had no way to combat internal infections. We just didn't have antibiotics in those days.

The diseases we face, as doctors, today are totally different. They are not the product of infection. Instead they are the result of subtle and unnatural forms of stress on the body over a number of years. They are lifestyle diseases, which need to be fought with lifestyle adjustments.

Our entire medical tradition (at least since

the turn of the century) is based on the idea of the search for the magic bullet...the particular pill that you can take to kill off the disease that is attacking your body.

But that idea no longer works.

No magic bullet will ever be found for heart disease, or diabetes, or cancer, or multiple sclerosis....or many other diseases. Because there are no bacteria or tiny bugs coming in from the outside and attacking your system.

You can't kill the disease-causing germ, in other words.

The "Law of 20 Years"

The real enemy is us. The things we do that get our bodies out of balance. It doesn't bother us at first. But after a few years, it begins to take its toll. In fact, this issue has been studied in great detail. T. L. Cleave, author of *The Sacchine Disease* (Keats, 1978), looked at the historical records to find out what happened when a formerly backward, or isolated, group abandoned its traditional eating habits and began to eat like you and I.

In particular, he singled out the people of Iceland, who switched to our diet in about 1920, and the nomadic Yemenite Jews who also made the switch. Previously, they ate very little sugar or refined carbohydrates and had no diabetes or atherosclerosis. It took twenty years after the switch was made for the first cases to appear.

But now, these groups have about the same incidence of modern ailments as we have.

From this evidence, Cleave developed the Rule of Twenty, meaning, it takes about 20 years before the effects of your lifestyle catch up to you.

There is so much evidence for this—a mountain of it actually—that there's not much room for debate.

The trouble is, it is very unsettling to the medical industry.

Everyone knows that these lifestyle diseases are, in fact, a by-product of modern life. And everyone knows that they creep up on you slowly over a period of years. And everyone also knows that small adjustments in your lifestyle can pay big rewards.

But most doctors know very little about the lifestyle treatments that you can use to prevent and reverse these problems. Such as nutritional antioxidants. Or acupuncture. Or food allergies. Chelation therapy. Or vitamins, minerals, and herbs. Or mineral transporters. In fact, they know almost nothing about nutrition. Period.

Yet these things are precisely where the big successes are coming from in the fight against modern disease.

"Heroic medicine" doesn't work

The model that most doctors use is completely inappropriate. It's like fighting WWII with a blunderbuss!

They are still looking for the magic bullet. And since there are no magic bullets in this fight...they offer various drugs to cover up the illness, to disguise the symptoms, or substitute one problem for another one.

Doctors are trained to intervene heroically to save lives by taking bold, decisive action. Attacking the problem... fighting the germs... destroying the bacteria—Magic Bullets—even the words are bold and forceful.

I like to be a hero too. As much as any doctor. But modern illnesses just don't care. You can administer all the drugs and do all the surgery you want. It barely has any effect. Chemotherapy, for example, is usually a waste of time (not to mention painful to the patient). Statistically, the life expectancy of a patient getting chemotherapy and not getting chemotherapy is about the same.

My patients aren't in those statistics. Because I've found that by concentrating on building up the patient's immune system and correcting the fundamental imbalance in the patient's system, we can greatly improve on the statistics. In fact, usually, we can turn this deadly disease into a manageable condition that the patient can live with indefinitely.

If Mrs. Onassis had tried Complementary Medicine first . . .

That's why I was saddened a few years ago

when I read in the paper about the death of Jacqueline Kennedy Onassiss. Rather than attempt to build up the patient's underlying health...or manage the disease...the attending physicians decided to go for broke with heavy chemotherapy. They were going to kill it or kill her. This is typical heroic doctor practice. Think like General "Blood and Guts" Patton. Seek and destroy. Go in with everything you've got to try to gain a decisive victory. The trouble is, unfortunately, it rarely works. Unfortunately, Mrs. Onassis died. Complementary medicine could have given her more choices.

No doctor likes to second guess a colleague. Jackie Onassis got the best care that that model of medicine provides. I have no quarrel with the doctors who provided the care. They did what they had been taught to do. And they did it, no doubt, very well. The trouble is with the model itself.

Forget Patton

What has to happen to win this fight is for the doctor to take off his battle gear and team up with the patient to find solutions.

Yes, there are solutions. Many of them. I've seen patients that were incurable. But I've never seen an ailment that couldn't be cured...or, at least, substantially alleviated.

The key is to work with the patient to find the real problem...re-establish the correct balance...and build up the patient's general health. This can be done to an astonishing degree.

But it requires an approach that is totally alien to most doctors...and generally disliked by the American Medical Association. Happily, in the meantime, people are getting well. Let me introduce you to a few of them.

Chapter 6

Healing Diabetes, and Hypoglycemia

"I improved on the low-carbohydrate diet almost immediately. The change was like night and day. It's truly unbelievable. I find myself feeling stronger and I can focus better. I know I'm on the right track."

Marian Peck

Marian's story illustrates about 95% of all the diabetics we see at the Atkins Center. It is a typical example of adult-onset diabetes, and how it's so often mistreated by orthodox medicine.

When Marian first went to her doctor complaining of fatigue and low energy, she was told she had a diabetic tendency. Her doctor prescribed the typical diet recommended by the American Diabetes Association.

Within two weeks she felt worse.

Not surprising, when you consider that the ADA diet is the complete opposite of what diabetics need to control their disease. The ADA diet is high in calories and carbohydrates, which only add fuel to the fire.

Remember. Your body turns carbohydrates into glucose—which demands insulin. And if you have a diabetic tendency, your body is most likely already producing too much insulin.

The road to recovery

A glucose tolerance test confirmed Marian's diabetes in addition to candidiasis. I started her on my low-carbohydrate diet and a supplement program that included many of the break-through natural therapies, like taurine and glutathione, I told you about earlier.

Within a few months, Marian's glucose reached a nearly normal 124. Her blood pressure fell from 160/92 to 140/80. Her fatigue vanished and she felt energized enough to take on the world.

I have seen patient after patient on the low-carbohydrate diet make incredible strides like Marian. Yet, physicians continue to push precisely the wrong diet.

I have treated hundreds of patients with Type II diabetes who were put on low-fat, high-carbohydrate diets and consequently ended up on insulin to cope with the high glucose levels that resulted. Physicians simply don't know enough about nutrition.

Every one is at risk

Let's take another look at the effects of unstable blood sugar levels. As I explained in Chapter 3, our bodies are not equipped to deal with the excessive quick-energy, simple-sugar, 20th-century diet.

Most people today are unable to handle the excess glucose of a high-carbohydrate, high-sugar diet. Their bodies overreact, causing a rapid rise in glucose, followed by its swift, prolonged fall because of an excess of insulin. This reaction is called hypoglycemia, or reactive hypoglycemia (RHG).

Symptoms include:

- ❑ fatigue
- ❑ depression
- ❑ dizziness
- ❑ irritability
- ❑ irregular heartbeat
- ❑ sugar cravings
- ❑ eating disorders
- ❑ jitteriness
- ❑ "brain fog"
- ❑ headache
- ❑ panic attacks
- ❑ alcohol cravings
- ❑ caffeine cravings

While these symptoms may seem minor at first glance, they can be life threatening.

I had one patient who suffered for 20 years with constant fatigue. He had been to a half dozen doctors before coming to see me. In less than a week on my low-carbohydrate diet, his symptoms disappeared. A few weeks later, he ate a plateful of pasta and bread at a dinner meeting, and afterwards, driving home alone, stopped for a red light. The next thing he knew a policeman was waking him up. The fatigue induced by his meal knocked him out in the middle of traffic. Fortunately, it didn't result in an accident.

Orthodox medicine won't admit to this troubling condition

Mainstream medicine is hell-bent on ignoring the existence of RHG. They insist that it is too rare to diagnose. They refuse to conduct the five-hour glucose tolerance test that has been used successfully since 1924. As a result, thousands of patients have gone misdiagnosed.

Another patient of mine, Barbara Lynch, suffered for over 20 years from repeated fainting spells, especially if she skipped meals. This should have been a dead giveaway to any doctor that she was hypoglycemic, but she was misdiagnosed over and over again. She also suffered from migraines, insomnia, irritable bowel syndrome, leg cramps, mood swings, and constant hunger and sugar-cravings.

Over the years, Barbara has had several glucose tolerance tests that turned out normal. A couple years ago, though, she finally had a proper GTT that proved she had hypoglycemia. We put her on the standard low-carbohydrate diet with supplements. Within 3 weeks her symptoms were improved.

Barbara has been symptom-free for almost two years

"The longer I'm on my diet," she says, *"the better I feel."*

If hypoglycemia is left undiagnosed and untreated long enough, the body will lose its ability to supply enough insulin or to employ the insulin it produces, resulting in high blood-sugar levels and the early stages of diabetes.

How to avoid the glucose rollercoaster ride

This vicious cycle, which may already have begun in you, must be counteracted and put to rest.

I have seen at least 15,000 patients with abnormal GTTs (hypoglycemic and diabetic) and over 99% showed improvement on the low-carbohydrate diet. It can happen almost overnight, just by switching from eating the wrong foods to eating the right foods.

Take John Parlone, for example. At 58 he was diagnosed as a Type II diabetic in the early stages. He was a big sweets eater with a passion for cake.

Within two months on a low-carbohydrate diet, John's blood pressure, which had been dangerously high for nearly a decade, dropped to 140/80 and he lost over 20 pounds. Within 3 months, his diabetes was under control and we were able to discontinue his medication. In less than a year, we got his blood pressure down to 116/70, he lost 35 more pounds, his cholesterol dropped from 296 to 251, and his triglyceride levels fell from 187 to 77.

John is a textbook case. But I've seen hundreds of others just like his. All it takes are some simple dietary changes and supplements to get the body back in balance and free your life of disease.

Chapter 7

Cures for the Heart: Hypertension, Atherosclerosis, Congestive Heart Failure, Heart Attack

---

" Within months, Dr. Atkins helped me turn my life around. I wasn't tired all the time, I didn't have to worry about the side-effects of drugs, and I didn't have to starve on a low-fat diet."
Patrick McCarthy

Patrick McCarthy is a 55-year-old teacher who first felt the indications of heart disease on vacation a few years ago.

Naturally, he went to the doctor, who prescribed the common beta blocker propranolol. The result was total exhaustion. Later he was put on verapamil, and when further testing revealed no improvement, the dosages were doubled. Patrick saw no end in sight. Finally, in the fall of 1989, he came to see me at the Atkins Center.

We restricted his diet to regulate his sugar/ insulin levels and gave him the standard nutrients for the heart.

Within four months he was off his medication. A recent stress test has shown indications of *reversal* of the blockages in his major arteries. His chest pain has not returned, and *all* of his risk factors for heart disease have reversed.

Is this man on a bleak, restrictive diet?

Listen. Patrick has a two-egg cheese omelet for breakfast each morning, sometimes with filet mignon. He has chicken, beef, or fish with a salad or vegetables at lunch, and his portions are large. At dinner he'll have a large steak, lamb chops, a pot roast, or a beef stew with plenty of vegetables. He likes broccoli with cheese and salads with blue cheese dressing. For dessert he'll have diet Jello. When snacking, macadamia nuts are his favorite.

Such austerity! Such suffering!

Naure's most luxurious foods . . . are also her most powerful healing tools

I know what you're thinking. Such a diet couldn't possibly be good for the heart.

Of course, what else are you supposed to believe? You've been constantly bombarded with conventional propaganda telling you that the diet I've seen work near miracles for patients is bad for your heart. You've had the opposite message drummed into your head so repetitively that you know with certainty that eating cream and butter and red meat causes heart attacks. That it will make your heart symptoms worse.

Don't believe it.

Good food is good for your heart too!

Certainly more beneficial for your heart than the sugar-laden, overprocessed, low-fat diet being pushed today.

I've seen the benefits almost from the first moment I began using the low-carbohydrate diet over 25 years ago.

✓ Patients with chest pain found their angina clearing up, often within days of going on the diet.

✓ Patients with episodes of cardiac arrhythmias maintained a normal rhythm as long as they kept to the diet.

✓ Patients with hypertension lowered their blood pressure—and fast.

Mary Campbell, for example, came to me a month after being hospitalized with a hypertensive crisis. She was suffering relentlessly from the side effects of her drug therapy.

Within six weeks of following my low-carbohydrate diet and time-tested nutritional supplements Mary was off all of her debilitating medications. Her blood pressure readings were below 130/84. After 10 weeks she regained her energy and all her lab values returned to normal.

The cholesterol myth

The faulty preconception that a low-carbohydrate diet should, by rights, be heart hazardous is based on a knee-jerk linguistic reaction to the words fat and cholesterol.

Forget what has been drummed into your head. Only a small part of North America's popular obsession with cholesterol now has any scientific validity.

It's not the amount of cholesterol we eat that counts. It's the amount of cholesterol that our bodies manufacture and the amount that becomes a certain kind of cholesterol that lends itself to building up on the insides of arteries.

What I'm saying is a little shocking. But it's true.

Cholesterol is necessary for survival

And studies prove this.

People with very low blood cholesterol readings die before people whose levels are in the 160 to 220 range. They're more vulnerable to cancer, emphysema, suicide and alcoholism, studies have documented, and they're more likely to meet violent deaths.

What's most important is the ratio of cholesterol. You want to shoot for high levels of HDL (the good cholesterol). The higher the ratio of HDL to LDL (the bad cholesterol), the better protected against heart disease you become.

You *can* reverse heart disease— permanently

The amazing benefit of my nutrition program is that patients are able to not only lower their risks, but they can actually *reverse* damage already done. If they stick to the program, they can maintain their lower levels *permanently*. Low-fat diets just don't work—or work long enough—to permanently reduce cholesterol.

They may lower cholesterol for the short-term, say, several months, but after six months cholesterol climbs back up, returning to or often exceeding the original point (*The American Journal of Clinical Nutrition*, 1991, 53:1404-1410).

My program's stabilizing effect on blood sugar helps control heart rhythm. By minimizing the rise and fall of glucose levels, the diet eliminates the body's need to use the heart stimulant adrenaline to raise quickly falling blood sugar.

Michael Shepard's arrhythmia virtually vanished—without drugs

One patient of mine, Michael Shepard, began suffering from heart arrhythmia when he was 14. His doctors sent him home on drug therapy, with a host of side effects, including exhaustion and hallucinations. Of course, he wasn't given any dietary advice, just the beta blocker propranolol.

When Michael came to see me, I immediately administered a glucose tolerance test. Michael's blood sugar went from 82 to 176 in the first hour, but over the next two hours dropped to 31! He definitely had a blood sugar problem.

I immediately started him on my no sugar diet and prescribed a basic supplement program along with magnesium orotate, L-glutamine, and additional B vitamins.

Within a few months, Michael's heart rhythm was perfect.

Over 90 percent of our patients have been able to discontinue, or at least reduce, their heart medication burden by following a low-carbohydrate diet with a tailored supplement program.

Ed Weaver *reversed* his heart disease through diet alone!

Ed progressed from a coronary angiogram (the invasive kind) that showed many artery blockages, to a noninvasive angiogram showing <u>better than normal function only a year later</u>. This is documentation of <u>heart disease reversal of a greater magnitude than I have ever seen before</u>.

Ed came to me in 1980, shortly after his fiftieth birthday. He was so exhausted he could barely walk around the block. He suffered frequent bouts of depression and was just plain miserable.

His cardiologist had him on four different drugs, all of which lead to his debilitating symptoms. I immediately weaned him off the clofibrate and reduced his other medications. I placed him on a personalized version of the Atkins low-carbohydrate diet and prescribed nutritional supplements, including extra magnesium orotate, B15, lecithin, vitamin E, zinc, manganese, selenium, garlic, and cod-liver oil at bedtime.

Within 6 months, Ed's cholesterol dropped over 100 points, his triglycerides fell from 196 to 93, and he lost 50 pounds. A year later, Ed's treatments had him *"feeling like a new man."*

Cardiologists turn their patients into drug addicts

Ed is typical of all too many coronary insufficiency patients, who are suffering as much from their medications as from their illness. His dramatic improvement as he gradually shed his medication burden is typical of hundreds.

The emphasis in orthodox prevention still remains on using drugs to reduce blood pressure, to prevent rhythm disorders, to prevent platelet clumping, to control heart rate, to lower lipid concentrations, to lessen the blood flow to the heart.

The net result is that patients often come in for a reevaluation of their heart management program suffering more from their medications than from their underlying disorder. We've seen thousands of patients like that at the Atkins Center.

Diuretics, the most widely prescribed category of drugs, are known to disturb sugar metabolism, raise uric acid, cholesterol, and triglyceride levels, and subject patients to heart rhythm disturbances.

And the beta blockers, currently the alternate No. 2 choice, cause so much depression that most patients prescribed beta blockers are also prescribed antidepressants.

All of this, when heart disease can be beaten via nutrition.

No effect of carbohydrate restriction is better documented than the fact that it consistently has a diuretic effect and causes an immediate salt and water loss. My patients are often surprised to see how many more trips to the bathroom they take just forty-eight hours after being on the program.

This water-excreting effect makes the diet fundamental therapy for both hypertension and congestive heart failure, two conditions for which diuretics are typically used. The most often confirmed medical fact in all my practice experience is the blood-pressure-lowering effects of any low-carbohydrate diet.

Chelation as a mainstay

Let's look at another case history. This time, I also prescribed chelation, one of my mainstays in treating heart disease.

Margaret Hare came to me when she was 62 and looking a great deal older.

Margaret had been diagnosed with angina and hypoglycemia. She had already suffered a coronary. She was immediately placed on drug therapy, including 3 nifedipine, 3 Corgard, and 3 Isordil tablets daily. She was regularly fed nitroglycerine through a skin patch.

"I was on so many drugs, I was like a zombie. I couldn't take care of myself," she says.

A year after her coronary and drug therapy, Margaret felt no better. That's when she came to see me.

I placed her on a low-carbohydrate diet with

antioxidants, garlic, magnesium orotate, bromelain, lecithin, zinc, and others. We gradually cut back on her medications, and within a few months we began chelation therapy.

After a year, Margaret's angina was markedly improved. For the first time in years, she was able to go out alone and do Christmas shopping. All of her symptoms diminished and her blood pressure had normalized.

"You cannot believe the difference. When I first arrived, I couldn't carry my pocketbook. My family didn't think I was going to live. Now I feel like a totally new person. I no longer think about death or life. I just live."

Margaret has not only had years of life, she has had years of good health.

I have used chelation therapy on more than a thousand of my heart patients like Margaret, and about 85 percent of them have improved. Chelation's effectiveness allows me to claim confidently that heart disease can be *reversed*.

Chapter 8

Health Frauds and Medical Rip-Offs

Though the model most doctors follow is woefully inadequate to deal with modern health problems...that doesn't stop them from trying. There's a lot of professional pride, prestige, and billions of dollars at stake.

Working hand in glove with the drug industry, they develop treatments that are then certified by various medical boards and doled out to patients as though they were aspirin.

Some of these treatments are just ineffective. Others are dangerous. All are expensive.

But all suffer from the same basic problem—the idea that nature must be defeated. When a person has a health problem, the mainstream view is that something has gone wrong in nature...and must be fixed. It's really not much different from fixing a car. If you have a runny nose...it's as if a car had a leak in a radiator hose. The drug industry would set to work on something that would stop the leak.

They would have no way of knowing what long term damage might be done...as long as the nose stopped running...the treatment would be deemed a success.

Or suppose you had diarrhea, a fever, or you gained weight...or you had a tumor? No matter what the problem, the idea would be to stop it...to cut it out...to fix whatever was going wrong.

Thus, the drugs that are used are most often designed to prevent your body from doing what it wants to do...to defeat nature, in other words.

But nature has been around for a much longer time than pharmaceutical companies or the AMA. And trying to defeat it is a losing proposition.

Rather than take the easy way out . . . I dig even deeper

If you have the symptom of a disease, you should pay attention to it. And instead of trying to block it or stop it or suppress it, the thing to do is to find out what it means. Then, instead of fighting against the symptoms, it's much more effective to bring the body's systems back in balance with nature...build up your overall health...making you stronger, healthier. Then, the symptoms go away all by themselves. Because you've corrected the underlying cause.

Instead, the majority of the medical profession has charged off in the wrong direction. And, in the process, they've created some of the biggest frauds and rip-offs in medical history.

Two hundred years ago, doctors got the idea that the way to help a sick person was to bleed him. The illness was in the blood, they reasoned, and bleeding would get it out of the system. George Washington survived years in the wilderness, he survived the French and Indian War...and survived the American Revolution. But even he couldn't survive this treatment! It killed him in 1799.

Even during our own lifetimes, we've seen such wrongheaded fads. Remember in the 50s when doctors removed childrens' tonsils at the drop of a hat? Now we know that was a mistake. But doctors continue to do things just as wrongheaded.

The campaign against cholesterol

The national campaign against cholesterol practically destroyed the egg business. But, is there any reason not to eat eggs? None whatsoever.

The myth that eggs are somehow linked with heart disease received its impetus fifty years ago when research sponsored by the Cereal Institute (please do notice the sponsor) demonstrated that feeding eggs to animals and humans would raise their serum cholesterol level.

However, as Bruce Taylor, M.D., of Albany Medical College in New York, pointed out that all the compelling research of the early years was done by feeding dried egg yolk powder, not fried or poached eggs, as eggs are usually eaten. Then he proved that the dried yolk powder is an oxidized form that is toxic to the blood vessels. This would make all of the early powdered egg yolk studies worthless. But orthodox medicine did not listen. And cholesterol was still seen as the enemy of the heart. (*American Journal of Clinical Nutrition,* vol. 32, 1979.)

Wrong, Wrong, Wrong

There are now close to a dozen published studies showing very little, if any, cholesterol elevation from eating eggs.

In fact, eggs are among the most nutritious of foods. Eggs, along with roe, plant seeds, and sprouts, are germinative foods. These foods, by nature's design, contain all the essentials for the growth of an organism.

The cholesterol content of eggs is actually offset by their considerable content of lecithin, itself a very good cholesterol-lowering agent. Further, the egg is considered the ideal protein source, containing the amino acids in the closest thing to a perfect ratio. Eggs are especially high in the sulfur-containing amino acids (cysteine, methionine, taurine), which are among the most clinically useful nutrients.

The amino acid L-cysteine is needed by the body to make glutathione. Glutathione is one of our more powerful antioxidants. It helps all of the other antioxidants in your body to slow cancer, prevent cataracts, prevent the oxidation of LDL cholesterol, and slow aging. It is also vitally important in the nutritional control of viruses.

The other sulfur-containing amino acid is L-methionine. It's required for the body to produce S-adenosyl methionine, which research shows is useful in treating osteoarthritis, Parkinson's disease, and chronic fatigue syndrome.

Your body also needs methionine to make taurine, a nutrient almost indispensable in the natural treatment of water retention, tissue swelling, macular degeneration, seizures, and heart failure.

That's why I regularly urge my patients to eat eggs.

And look at the other health benefits. Lecithin is also a natural emulsifier. It helps liquefy fat inside the blood vessels and prevent buildups from blocking arteries. Lecithin is the body's major phospholipid, a kind of fat that is essential to keeping cell membranes fluid. Fluidity prevents cells from aging and may possibly help preserve the regular rhythm of the heart.

The simple truth is, unless you're among the 2 percent of people who are allergic to egg yolks, you have nothing to fear. So enjoy...with my blessing.

The low-fat food fraud

Or, take the low-fat food craze...or the whole idea of low-fat diets.

The medical industry...and the food industry...have gone for this hook, line and sinker. What's the real story?

The low-fat, high-carbohydrate diet is responsible for the one-diet-fits-all health disaster plaguing the public today. The evidence of the failure of the low-fat diet is pouring in. But the

---

Only 3%-5% of dieters on the low fat program lose weight and keep it off. The low-fat diet doesn't work. Period. Case closed.

---

consensus refuses to look at it.

As I predicted many years ago, for many people, eating pasta, bread, grains, fruits, and other carbohydrates is self-defeating. It'll thicken their waistlines, envelop them in a fog of fatigue, and shove them face first into the consequences of heart disease and diabetes.

While the establishment authorities applaud the national reduction of fat intake—down from more than 40% of total calories to 33%—they scratch their heads at the inescapable consequences: In the last 10 years, 20 million people in the United States became defined as obese, and the number of obese children doubled. The average American put on 10 pounds in the last decade.

The very authorities responsible for this new epidemic refuse to shoulder the blame, preferring to attribute the national belly bulge to a

They're WRONG about...

1 **Heart disease and eggs**: I've been putting my heart patients on high-egg diets for years...and, guess what! They actually show <u>impressive gains in the heart-protecting good HDL cholesterol</u>. Recent studies support what I have long known to be fact. Get the truth! (Turn to page 65)

They're WRONG about...

2 **Diabetes and the high-carbohydrate diet**: For decades, diabetics have been told to chain themselves to a diet low in fat and high in rice, pasta, and breads. I've known for decades that this diet is MURDER for a diabetic! I've found a <u>breakthrough program</u> that can wean most type II diabetics off their medication! (Turn to page 47)

They're WRONG about...

3 **Migraines and food allergies**: While orthodox medicine has been known to tinker with food allergies when trying to find a cure for migraines...I've found it isn't always dairy or chocolate that triggers the pounding. (Turn to page 85 to see how one woman replaced her narcotic pain killers with my <u>simple</u> nutrient program!)

They're WRONG about...

4 **Arthritis and unproven remedies**: A few years ago the Arthritis Foundation published a pamphlet that warned you to be suspicious of doctors who treat your arthritis with nutrition! Over 20 years ago, I began putting together an anti-arthritic supplement program...and today that program alone helps 92% of my patients significantly reduce if not completely eliminate their medication. (Turn to page 81)

They're WRONG about...

5 **Cancer and chemotherapy**: While cancer specialists all over the world are trying to poison the tumor or cancer cells out of existence...I've been turning my practice towards the <u>causes</u> of immune system breakdown. <u>Every day I discover new ways of combining nutrients and botanicals to build UP your immune system</u>. (See page 73 to discover the nutrients that give the most tremendous near-miraculous results!)

lack of exercise (in the midst of a boom in the fascination with fitness) and to the sudden desire to eat uninhibitedly. Not a shred of evidence exists to support such contentions. They are unable (or unwilling) to recognize the obvious cause-and-effect relationship. Low-fat eating *causes* the epidemic.

There are no missing facts

By definition, the low-fat diet is a high-carbohydrate diet. It's the only food group left. Although fat consumption is down, carbohydrate consumption is up—by a 50 fattening grams a day. Simple science shows that carbohydrates—and only carbohydrates—increase the body's secretion of insulin.

And as I've said before, the overproduction of this hormone, along with the inherent inability of most of us to use it, is the prime cause of obesity, diabetes, and heart disease.

If you do what they say, you're taking risks with your health—serious risks that can lead to grave illness.

At the very least, you're cheating yourself out of ener_y and good health TODAY. At worst, you're robbing yourself of 10...even 20 years of a full, active rich life.

Why listen to me? After all, I'm telling you to <u>do the exact opposite</u> of what the AMA, the AHA, the FDA, the ADA...and most every other major health association in America is telling you to do.

How could one man be right, and everyone else be wrong?

To that reasonable question, I can only answer this:

I've been practicing medicine for over 30 years. I've helped over 60,000 patients recover their health often when other doctors—mainstream *and* alternative—had failed.

I followed my gut back in the 1960s, when I began working with the low-carbohydrate diet (contrary to what everyone else was doing)...and I've been following it ever since in my clinic in New York, patient by patient, illness by illness, recovery by recovery.

Instead of switching from fad to fad, I've stayed with the same proven health program for decades making changes, additions, improvements, and adjustments along the way. That's what the Atkins Center is all about: proven, solid, careful medicine designed to make you healthy without drugs, without surgery, without struggle.

Chapter 9

Dozens of Ways to Control Cancer

There is no better example of the weaknesses of orthodox medicine than it's clearly ineffective War on Cancer. Traditional cancer specialists have very little treatment options to offer. Either cut the cancer out, poison it with chemotherapy, or kill the cells with radiation. At the same time, they jeopardize the health of their patients by weakening their immune systems and compromising their self-healing resources.

I've been developing my own complementary cancer-treatment approach since the early 1980s. I've found that there is no better example of the superiority of a complementary approach than in the management of this dread disease.

Despite what you must think...

Cancer is a controllable illness

But you have to support the body fully, making it stronger so it can fight the cancer.

I've seen scores of cases in which cancer patients were getting worse, as indicated by blood tests. They came to me looking for hope. My complementary approach gave them just that, and more. I was able to help them help themselves improve dramatically using the nontoxic medicines standard to my treatment.

Denton Brill's story, which I told you about at the start of this book, illustrates this well. After getting Denton on a health-enhancing diet, you'll remember that I prescribed an antioxidant program that included an array of vitamins, minerals, and herbs.

Creating an ideal environment

Nutrition and botanicals are key to fighting cancer. For complementary cancer therapy to work, the immune system must be relatively intact. The biologic therapies work *through* the immune system; they cannot create a new one.

Rather than directing my entire arsenal on killing the tumor, I make sure the body is strong enough to hold its own. Then, I emphasize the substances that selectively make the tumor die while allowing normal, healthy cells and tissues to live. This is something orthodox treatments are completely unable to do.

To the immune system, chemotherapy is a disaster and a half. The inescapable conclusion is that even when chemotherapy works, alternatives must be considered.

Let's look at **Ukrain**, for example. This is probably the single best anticancer agent I use.

This substance, derived from celandine and thiophosphoric acid, is a safe, supportive alternative to chemotherapy. Given by injection, it kills tumor cells while fortifying the immune system. I've seen a 93% remission rate with patients who started treatment when the cancer was in its earliest stage.

The patented remedy **Carnivora**, derived from the Venus flytrap, also appears to work by lessening the malignant characteristic of the tumor, rather than by destroying tissue. This common German cancer remedy was developed by Helmut Keller, M.D. Among 210 of Dr. Keller's patients with terminal cancer, 34 went into remission and 84 showed a halt in disease progression after using Carnivora.

You should think of cancer as a tug of war between the patient and the disease. You need the *power pullers* on your side—natural substances that help the body destroy the cancer, usually by strengthening the immune system.

Another one of the strongest power pullers in my injectable arsenal is **714X** This substance, developed by Canadian biologist Gaston Naessens, is made from nitrogen-rich camphor and appears to neutralize a factor produced by tumor cells that ordinarily paralyzes the immune system. In other words, it doesn't kill the cancer cells directly, but blocks their feeding mechanism.

Orthodox medicine just doesn't get it

The exciting concept that mainstream oncologists do not grasp is that these are *nontoxic approaches* and that *the benefit-to-risk ratio is nearly "infinity."* Therefore, there is no reason not to combine dozens of them into a single patient program.

Which is what I aim to do in every case, using the Hippocratic pecking order. I gather as much data as possible on each patient and then do the safest of the effective things first and save the riskiest for last. Many of my patients do very well on the nontoxic therapies alone.

Building Chester's allied forces

Chester Delmas has been a ray of sunshine in the lives of all the staff at the Atkins Center. When he first came to see me, Chester had already had two surgeries to remove tumors from his colon and lung. His surgeon had recommended additional chemotherapy "as preventive medicine." He was sure he wanted nothing to do with chemotherapy.

I explained to Chester that there are two ways to win a battle. One is to weaken the enemy; the other is to build the allied forces. When I told him we would give him only agents that would build him up, the apprehension left his face.

Chester's lab tests looked like anything but those of a cancer patient. He had high cholesterol and his blood sugars even had that high-low pattern. His immune profile and tumor markers of all kinds were quite normal. His only medication was a beta blocker, and he was moderately overweight. I really had to treat him more like a blood pressure patient. I certainly wouldn't even consider chemotherapy as a "preventive."

Accordingly, I put him on an antioxidant program, including high dosages of vitamin C, natural beta carotene, vitamin E, selenium, coenzyme Q10, pycnogenol, N-acetyl cysteine, glutathione, and lipoic acid.

Employing the full spectrum of antioxidants is part of every Atkins Center patient's program, whether as treatment or prevention. They help protect cells' genetic material and membranes from free-radical damage, thereby preserving the cells' normal functions.

In addition to the antioxidants, I started Chester on primrose oil, germanium sesquioxide, pancreatic enzymes, thymus and liver extracts, plus our usual antihypertensive protocol.

Pancreatic enzymes are perhaps the most valuable of the oral supplements I use. These enzymes digest away the protective protein coating or shell that encases tumors, leaving the cancer cells vulnerable.

We also stopped his beta blocker and started him on intravenous vitamin C, with ozone, peptides from liver and spleen, and a program of mistletoe. Preparations made from fermented mistletoe have been used effectively by doctors in Germany for cancer treatment since 1920.

Today, all of Chester's tumor markers and immune profiles remain well within the normal range. His treatment has remained uneventful.

Chester's treatment only incorporated a small percentage of the nontoxic cancer treatments available. I'm sure you've heard of shark cartilage. The tough, elastic connective tissue from sharks seems to prevent cancer tumors from developing new blood vessels and expanding their blood supply.

Anyone interested in alternative cancer treatments should also know about the herbal formula Essiac. Given as a tea, Essiac's main components include slippery elm, burdock, Indian rhubarb, and sorrel. It is known to strengthen the immune system, reduce drug toxicity, enhance energy, and sedate inflammation. The herbs cats claw and Siberian ginseng are also potent anticancer substances, among others.

* * * * * * * * *

Now here is a very important footnote to all of this. Almost every one of these valuable health boosters is available right now, without prescription. They're safe. They're natural. Take them without risk or worry.

You can wait until you get sick...and they can help restore you to health. Or, you can begin taking them now. Make them part of your everyday life.

I'll show you what we've learned about them already...and keep you up-to-date as we discover more.

* * * * * * * * *

Perhaps the most important factor of all in fighting cancer is the right attitude. My regimen aims to enhance the patient's mood, attitude, and psychological state as a means of facilitating the healing process and to avoid producing anxiety, depression, or despair, which commonly occur under conventional care.

My staff and I expect the patient to get well and stay well. The power of this positive thinking is contagious. Cancer *survivors* do not give in to the intimidation and mental toxicity of conventional medicine.

The happy irony in complementary cancer treatment is that there are 3 or 4 new therapies in the pipeline that appear sufficiently promising that they may one day make the entire Atkins Center program outmoded.

Chapter 10

Easy Solutions to Ailments Most Doctors Can't Cure: Arthritis, Headaches, Candida, Irritable Bowel Syndrome

---

"When I first came to you, I could hardly walk. Now I don't think about it, I just walk without pain. I can even lift and use my right arm."

Maria Diamonte

Look at Maria Diamante. Maria came to the Atkins Center as a 55-year-old victim of **rheumatoid arthritis**. After a number of surgical procedures and debilitating drug therapy, orthodox treatment failed in providing an effective treatment.

A glucose tolerance test indicated the probable cause of Maria's inflammation—unstable sugar/insulin levels with a carbohydrate metabolism gone awry.

Immediately, I started her on the low-carbohydrate diet, which also served to eliminate some widely implicated food intolerances. I also removed nightshades (tomatoes, potatoes, paprika, eggplant, green pepper, tobacco) from her diet, since they are known to aggravate arthritis. I'll bet Maria's doctors never told her about the nightshades. I also placed her on a supplement program and weaned her off the four different drugs she was taking.

Within six months Maria was a new woman.

Her doctors view her as a miracle

They can't believe how well and free of pain Maria is today.

If there is one single condition that can best be used to evaluate a system of medicine, it has to be arthritis. Arthritis provides enough chronicity and confusion to frustrate any doctor's attempt at healing. And, unfortunately, most doctors do fail to treat the *cause* of arthritis. Instead, they settle for masking its symptoms. Which is all that Maria's doctors were able to do for her when they prescribed aspirin, an NSAID, prednisone, and the diuretic hydrochlorothiazide.

Orthodoxy rarely digs deeper into causation than to recognize that arthritis is caused by inflammation. This leads to the use of anti-inflammatory agents, which admittedly are one step deeper into dealing with causation than are simple painkillers.

But what causes the inflammation?

If orthodox doctors took the time to get to the root of the cause, rather than focusing on pigeonhole diagnoses and symptoms, they would come to find that seemingly complex, multifaceted disorders, like arthritis, may have simple solutions.

My complementary approach concerns finding and correcting causation. In Maria's case it was a sugar disorder. The same causation can cause different problems in different people. I've found that most causation centers around our 20th-century diet and 20th-century environmental factors.

In the case of arthritic patients, as in so many others as well, we look for food intolerances, sugar disorders, heavy metal accumulations, yeast or parasitic overgrowth, and autoimmune reactivity. Once the causative factors have been identified, the hand plays itself.

Remove the cause of the imbalance and the patient gets better. It's that simple.

Bob Kelley was another success. All it took to cure him of arthritic knees was to identify his food sensitivities. It turned out that Bob was sensitive to nightshades, yeast, cheese, wheat, mushrooms, broccoli, carrots, oranges, and vinegar.

Within two weeks of avoiding these foods, Bob's pain disappeared, and it hasn't returned since.

Putting a halt to headache

As I pointed out earlier, often times the cause of one disease is the same as another. Just as the wrong diet and nutrition caused Bob's and Maria's arthritis, it is often the cause behind another growing epidemic—headache.

Headache is a symptom so prevalent and so debilitating that it has achieved disease status and has evoked the development of dozens of headache clinics. But, alas, the experience of headache-clinic caregivers has, in my opinion, provided very little real advantage for their patients.

Orthodox headache clinics fail to cure the *cause*. They overemphasize diagnostic testing, they almost totally refuse to consider dietary connections, they only offer pigeonhole diagnoses, and they invariably rely on drugs that only relieve symptoms.

I have treated more than a thousand patients complaining of frequent headaches, and have seen the headaches eradicated in over 90% of them. Not by a drug, or even a vitamin combination, but by prevention.

Our preventive precept is elementary: Find out what *causes* the headaches and stop doing it. And, like arthritis, the clues to causation most often lie in blood glucose dynamics or in the field of allergy/intolerance.

Hypoglycemia was the cause that lead to Roberta's relief

Roberta Stein came to me after suffering from migraines since she was 15. She had been seeing orthodox physicians, who essentially turned her into a drug addict. Our screening lab tests showed she was hypoglycemic. I immediately removed Roberta from all medication and put her on a strict low-carbohydrate diet with additional supplements.

A mere 10 days later, Roberta came back to me, and said, *"I feel fantastic. No headache. My energy is better. My sleep is better."*

After examining the facts of her case, I think it's safe to conclude that simply by regulating Roberta's blood sugar levels via the low-carbohydrate diet, we were able to eliminate her headaches.

That's not to say that a low-carbohydrate diet can ease everyone's headaches. It may be a simple food allergy. Caffeine, dairy products, chocolate, and wheat products are often the underlying cause of headaches. While your doctor may tell you to avoid caffeine or chocolate, most likely, they won't conduct the proper tests to rule out other possible culprits. Most people aren't just allergic to one food.

Overcoming IBS

Food allergies are clearly a common culprit as the cause of irritable bowel syndrome (IBS).

The greatest offender is wheat, followed by corn, dairy products and yeast.

The food allergy approach is fully ready for acceptance into the mainstream. But it has not been accepted. Mainstream specialists don't do food-allergy testing. Despite the fact that there are plenty of experimental studies published in peer-reviewed journals. Again, they would rather rely on treating symptoms, rather than the cause, with drugs.

Other solutions to IBS are found in diet and nutrition. Again, this is an area where the low-carb diet to regulate sugar/insulin levels is effective. Another common cause is a Candida albicans infection (yeast overgrowth). IBS is a common symptom of this underlying cause. In fact, Candida albicans overgrowth can also cause arthritic symptoms and actual food intolerances.

The Candida connection

There are so many symptoms of Candida that it usually goes undiagnosed. Instead, doctors end up treating the symptoms, which never seem to go away.

I can offer you at least two easy solutions to this seemingly incurable illness: cut your intake of sugar and/or eliminate antibiotics.

Just as the use of sugar, when added to yeast, helps make bread rise, so does sugar increase the effects of yeast in the body. Antibiotics, especially oral antibiotics, cause overgrowth of Candida albicans as well.

In addition to these solutions, a low-carbohydrate diet and a low-yeast diet that avoids the major food intolerances, like wheat and dairy, are beneficial. Of course, I never suggest any form of treatment without additional supplementation. In this case, I would emphasize beneficial bacteria to help rebuild the proper balance in the colon.

As you can see, all of these incurable ailments can be easily treated if they're approached in the right way in the first place. If doctors followed the complementary lead and aimed for the *cause*, rather than diagnosing the symptoms, these problems wouldn't be left uncured or even undiagnosed.

Chapter 11

How to Lose Weight Without Really Trying

My curiosity in trying to understand why some people gained weight and others didn't proved to be the foundation for an entirely new healing approach. The low-carbohydrate nutrition program really shows its merit against the very intractable...often "incurable"...modern illnesses.

The very reason why the low-carbohydrate diet works to cure and contain these modern illnesses goes back to our original insight behind the Atkins diet. These 20th century diseases didn't begin to surface in such number until after the introduction of sugar and highly refined, processed foods. Our bodies were not equipped to deal with the huge influx of sugar consumption—thus throwing our blood sugar/insulin levels out of wack. When you have a fundamental imbalance like this, things are bound to go wrong.

My diet restores this balance by regulating carbohydrate intake. The body converts carbohydrates into sugar, which adds fuel to the fire and upsets the sugar/insulin balance. In addition, I found that carbohydrates actually become addictive—resulting in a greater intake of calories.

Which leads to the bonus effect of my low-carbohydrate diet. Not only can it prevent and cure modern-day disease—it can help you lose weight. So while you're eating to prevent or reverse ill health, you can lose weight at the same time—without even trying.

Most people who are overweight have a metabolic imbalance. The basic principles of my diet actually work to restore a healthy balance to your natural metabolic system. Instead of starving my patients on a low-calorie diet, I concentrate on lowering the levels of carbohydrate consumption drastically so that fat can be burned off by a process called ketosis.

Mary Anne Evans ate all she wanted—and lost 70 lbs

One patient of mine, Mary Anne Evans, was able to lose 70 pounds, lower her blood pressure from 160/100 to 120/78, and overcome her fatigue with little effort. She had tried countless diets—low-calorie diets—including Weight Watchers; a hospital-based program that measured calories; and a liquid protein diet on which she lost more than thirty pounds in three months and gained it back, with interest in four.

Immediately, I had Mary Anne restrict her carbohydrates. She abandoned the crackers she ate with lunch and the potato she had with dinner, she gave up a few other things too, but some of them only temporarily.

So what did she eat? Ham and eggs for breakfast, tuna fish for lunch, and chicken, pork chops, or steak for dinner. Mary Anne lost 10 pounds in 16 days and her fatigue had gone. After five weeks, she'd lost 21 pounds, and her blood pressure was 120/78.

"It was so easy to do this," she said. *"I lost weight without any hassle...and I was never hungry."*

Now she eats two potatoes weekly and plenty of vegetables and salads. She's on a luxury diet, full of energy, and her blood pressure is normal.

How is this possible?

In the simplest terms, the diet causes weight loss by commanding the body to burn its own fat for fuel. In the body's energy-release pecking order, carbohydrate is the favored fuel. If there is very little carbohydrate in the diet, your body will dissolve its own fat, by liberating carbon fragments called ketones. This is where we get the term ketosis. When you are in a state of ketosis, you are burning fat!

This diet sets no limit on the amount of food you can eat, because it will naturally reduce your appetite for food. You will never be hungry again.

Let's look at Patricia Finley's menu. Patricia, who used to eat quite a lot of starches and who would sometimes go on massive dessert binges when she was under pressure, has converted to a tasty low-carbohydrate diet.

For breakfast, she eats bacon and eggs, or a cheese omelet, or some vegetables with blue cheese. Lunch can be tuna fish or chicken with a sumptuous salad. Sometimes, she'll have chopped sirloin, sauted with onions, chili powder and peppers. Patricia enjoys having olives or asparagus spears for snacks, but she puts the greatest amount of energy and attention into dinner. She finds that it isn't possible to feel deprived when you're enjoying guacamole and strips of chicken and steak. Add to that her passion for grated zucchini in olive oil with butter and nutmeg, her liking for broccoli with lemon butter sauce, and her homemade recipe for chicken soup. This is only a small sample of the food she finds it possible and delightful to eat on a diet!

What happens once you've lost the weight?

You keep it off, of course.

The Atkins nutrition program provides a permanent plan for maintaining ideal weight once your goal weight is reached. This is critical because, on most low-fat/ low-calorie diets, 95% of all dieters gain back the weight they've lost. (This is similar to the way my diet helps lower cholesterol levels permanently.) The Atkins diet lends itself to a lifetime maintenance diet that's suited to you.

To lose weight initially, you will not have to restrict your main courses, such as meat, fish, fowl, eggs, and cheese, but you'll have to restrict your carbohydrate intake. Once you've reached your ideal weight, you can gradually increase your carbohydrate intake slowly until you notice a slight weight gain. That's how you know when to stop and cut back a little.

The maintenance diet is a variation of the omnivorous diet our bodies were used to before the 20th century diet. You'll be eating meat, fish, fowl, eggs, vegetables, seeds and nuts to your heart's content. And you'll be eating fruits and whole grains to the extent your metabolism allows them without provoking weight regain.

So you can see now that the Atkins diet not only will help you achieve ideal health, but ideal weight as well. The fact that health and weight loss could be combined so perfectly together is something I don't foresee the medical establishment even coming close to as long as they hold on to their obsession with the low-fat/low-calorie diet.

For a complete explanation of my weight-loss diet, refer to my latest best-selling book, *Dr. Atkins' New Diet Revolution.* (See page 110 to find out how you can get this book at a special discounted rate.)

Here are some examples of the kinds of recipes I recommend to my patients:

Lemon Mousse
(12 servings)

7 eggs, separated, room temp.
1 1/2 cups heavy cream
juice from 3 large lemons

1 env. unsweet. gelatin
3 tbs orange cordial
6-10 packets of sugar substitute

Cream sweeteners and egg yolks. In a double boiler, combine lemon juice with gelatin and melt. When melted, dribble in sweetened egg yolks, stirring constantly. Set aside. Whip heavy cream. When stiff, fold in egg-gelatin mixture. Beat egg whites until peaks form. Fold into cream. Adjust sweetness. Cover with foil and let it set in refrigerator for several hours.
(Total grams carbohydrates: 19.2. Grams per serving: 1.6)

Warm Beef Salad
(8 servings)

16 oz cooked beef, shredded
8 oz raw mushroom caps, sliced
2 bunches watercress or arugula
1 tbs freshly grated horseradish

2 egg yolks
1 tbs red wine vinegar
4 tbs sesame oil
1 tbs toasted sesame seeds

Rinse watercress and dry thoroughly. Mix the vinegar and sesame oil. Pour over watercress and toss. Arrange the watercress on a plate. Mix the shredded beef, mushrooms, grated horseradish and egg yolks. Place the mixture on top of the watercress and sprinkle with the toasted sesame seeds.
(Total grams carbohydrates: 13.6. Grams per serving: 3.4)

Broccoli Fritata
(6 servings)

4 eggs
1 cup broccoli florets, cooked
1 large onion, thinly sliced
1/2 lb mushroom caps, thin sliced
1/2 tsp salt

1/2 tsp freshly ground pepper
4 tbs butter
3 tbs grated parmesan cheese
1 tsp baking soda
minced parsley, for garnish

Put 2 tbs butter in skillet. Saute onion and mushrooms until golden. Remove from heat. Put eggs, baking soda, salt and pepper into bowl and beat lightly. Add onion, mushrooms and broccoli. Mix well. Add remaining butter to skillet and pour in egg mixture. Fry on top of stove until eggs start to set. Sprinkle parmesan cheese on top and broil until golden. Remove from heat. Cut into wedges, garnish with parsley and serve. (Total grams carbohydrate: 31.2. Grams per serving: 5.2)

Chapter 12

Most Dreaded Diseases are Being Reversed

Given up as incurable, these people made spectacular comebacks after undergoing treatment at the Atkins Center for Complementary Medicine. They are all fully recovered. Here are their stories:

Angina pectoris eliminated

On a bright spring morning in 1991, Dom DeVito went digging in his garden and hit a nasty rock: rock bottom. He was trying to plant just one small azalea bush. But by the time he had dug six inches, he was exhausted. Panting and grasping his chest, he very slowly made his way back to the house, took a dose of beta blockers, and chewed on a celery stick, one of the few snacks his doctor allowed him.

The doctor was a pricey Park Avenue cardiologist who had watched him for 30 years and knew exactly what Dominic's problem was: a classic case of angina pectoris.

Like most angina victims, Dominic couldn't stand much exercise. He spent long hours with the TV and radio and fell asleep by eight o'clock almost every night, dead tired and in pain.

But one evening that year, Dom tuned in to WOR in New York and was still awake when my program came on. Encouraged by what he heard, he came to see me at the Atkins Center for Complementary Medicine. I gave him a prescription for an array of food supplements, and began chelation therapy.

Today he recalls: *"My cholesterol dropped even though I started eating lots of foods high in fat and cholesterol. After two months, I was able to start running again, something I hadn't done for years!*

After the third month, my chest pains stopped altogether, so I went out playing basketball regularly! One day I visited my old cardiologist. He was amazed at my recovery. But he thought it was his crummy diet and pills that had done it. So I told him about Dr. Atkins' methods. He was shocked and said, 'Why, you'll kill yourself!' I thought that was a pretty funny change of tone. I feel great!"

MS symptoms gone!

Diana Pinto has been on my program for multiple sclerosis for seven years. She fist came to me when her symptoms were out of control, with little energy and little hope. She felt she had nothing to lose.

"I found it hard to even walk the length of

the mall. I could not imagine being able to have a family—or even continuing my full time job.

Now, I have more energy than I thought would be possible. I haven't had a single setback since my first treatment. I have a daughter and son, ages four and two. I am working full time and pursuing my master's in business administration at night. I still have MS, but thanks to Dr. Atkins, I have found something that makes me strong to fight it.

I'm thankful he has brought this program over from Germany to give people a new chance. I don't worry about my MS getting worse anymore! The program—combined with vitamin therapy and more attention to nutrition—has allowed me to once again pursue my goals."

Heart disease reversed without surgery!

When Michael Levine came to see me, he was a walking time bomb. He was overweight, drank and smoked heavily, and had type II diabetes and high blood pressure.

The bomb finally went off in 1988 during a business trip. He suffered a heart attack, wound up in intensive care for two weeks, and was released with heavy medication and told by two doctors to get a bypass immediately. But he was too scared.

After reading my book, he came to see me at the Atkins Center. I immediately started him on L-carnitine and other nutrients, chelation therapy, and a tailored version of my low-carbohydrate diet.

"I was off all medication in one month. The heart problems are gone! I feel great, and very energetic."

Arthritis pain banished!

Study arthritis and you'll find two strange facts that separate it from other diseases: 1) Complementary Medicine has a greater number of effective treatments for it than for any other common condition, and yet... 2) The medical establishment bad-mouths every single one of them! For instance, the very-orthodox Arthritis Foundation has even published a list of remedies it does not think have any merit. Among them are vitamins, cod liver oil, homeopathy, acupuncture, herbs, and botanicals. But we regularly prescribe all of these for various patients—with significant improvement in movement and swollen joints almost every time.

When Faye Stern came to us in January of 1991, she was a sad sight indeed. Gnarled and in pain, she had insomnia, anemia, fatigue, and memory loss. Her sedimentation rate (the standard arthritic inflammation) was 138, compared to the normally acceptable 20. She had been on the powerful anti-inflammatary Prednisone.

We put her on a yeast-free diet based on meat and millet, and just one month later, she was able to start a modest exercise program.

Less than two years later, she has had no major flare-ups, she's quite active, and says, *"I feel fine!"*

What their stories mean to you

It wasn't easy for these patients to share their stories, but they share in the hope that they can help you and others find relief from your health problems. My staff and I help people like these every day. We know that each person and their problems are unique, and we want to help you.

If you or someone you know suffers from food-related illness and traditional medicine hasn't helped, don't give up. There are alternative therapies that could prove very effective and you can learn about them each month in my monthly newsletter *Health Revelations*.

Of course, keeping you healthy in the first place is our primary goal. To live a healthy and active live, to eat smart and maintain a balanced weight that is right for you, you need access to all the latest medical and nutritional information. I give that to you each month in *Health Revelations*.

Complementary Medicine is not incompatible with traditional medicine. It is the way to combine effective treatments from all valid medical practice to help you stay healthy. You will find explanations on the newest and most effective treatments each month in *Health Revelations*.

* * * * * * * * * *

And here's another very important point:

Since the time I wrote my first book, hundreds and thousands of doctors all over the world have begun to experiment with nutrition-based solutions and various forms of Complementary Medicine. There is now an explosion of new research, clinical findings, and real-life healing experience. We're coming up with new and better health solutions every day.

That is why it is so important to keep up with these breakthroughs. They can help you or someone you know, in a dramatic, even life-saving way.

My mission in publishing *Dr. Atkins' Health Revelations* is to bring this information to you so that you can put it to work in your life. Don't wait for the medical establishment to catch up— that could take decades!

* * * * * * * * * *

It's time you got serious about your health

Most of your friends are going to die far too soon. You, however, can probably avoid that fate...especially if you pay attention to the next few pages.

I'm going to tell you how to avoid ever having to sleep in a hospital bed, prove your gloom-

and-doom doctors wrong, and enjoy the kind of health that friends thirty years younger will envy.

I'm going to do all this by sending you a stream of privileged information that will allow you to sort out the true wisdom from the health misinformation you're being sold today.

This knowledge will cost you far less than 1% of the fortune you'll likely wind up paying to doctors and hospitals if you pass this by.

You're going to enjoy living a whole lot more—in a dozen ways. Your new life will begin as you take the following five steps.

1. Don't let drug companies and out-of-date doctors keep you in the dark! Open your eyes! Read the obituaries for a few days and see how the vast majority of your friends and neighbors are dying of diseases that have already been licked or controlled. Yet doctors who practice Complementary Medicine (regular physicians whose skills include most types of alternative treatments) treat successfully the very diseases that show up most often in your local obits.

Tradition-bound doctors are able to cure only about 25% of the ailments they treat! Most of what they do is relieve symptoms until your body's natural healing mechanisms and immune system can finish the job.

Think about how many people in your town are shut-in invalids, dependent on others, when they could be productive and living life to the fullest. Most people just expect to be bed-ridden eventually. How sad—and how unnecessary today.

You can't afford to drift along, depending on drugs and surgery, which is only half the medical care available. Break free from the herd! Light your own path! Your reward will be many extra years of life—and the physical freedom to enjoy it.

2. Expand your choices. Why let doctors play God in your life? Join the tiny minority who have decided to take charge of their own health. If you don't, you'll eventually find yourself trapped, like nine out of ten Canadians, in a living nightmare...

"I'm sorry," your doctor says somberly, *"but the results of your tests are conclusive. We must operate as soon as possible. We'll have to do a double bypass (or start chemotherapy, or remove your prostate, or do a hysterectomy, or whatever.)"*

You object, *"But isn't there something else we can do?"*

"No," he shakes his head, *"this is the way it's done. You have no choice."*

My experience with patients has taught me that such a statement is almost always wrong. You may have some very good choices. But he probably won't be familiar with them—or inclined to use them. And time may be pressing. You may not have a few weeks to research your options.

That's how millions of people will be trapped

this year: a sudden pain, a surprise symptom, and BINGO—there they are in the doctor's office, squirming like a hooked trout.

You probably think I'm trying to scare you. Well, maybe I am, a bit. But believe me, life itself often looks scary when you sit and talk to frightened people eight hours a day, people who never took charge of their own health, but just ate and behaved like all their friends and hoped for the best.

That's suicide by lifestyle, friend. Don't copy them!

3. Find a doctor who offers the full spectrum of treatments. You may now have a doctor with the highest reputation in your state.

But if he restricts himself to "orthodox" or "conventional" medicine alone, he is running on one cylinder instead of eight.

You need someone who knows his or her way around the block, someone who knows many types of therapies for every common disease; is responsible to you, not his peers or his hospital; isn't hypnotized by drug company claims—and conned by their constant barrage of gifts to doctors; has the guts to prescribe a course of treatment for you that may differ from "consensus opinion;" always tries to uncover the cause of your problem, not just the diagnosis; uses the safest therapies first; and knows which safe and natural therapies will complement your treatment.

Where can you find such a "dream doctor?" Here and there. You may have to travel out of your area, but they do exist.

4. Let nature work for you, not against you. Don't try to play tricks on Mother Nature. It's not very smart.

You'll soon find that she has her own tricks, and if you keep annoying her, she'll get even with you!

Stay on her side. Stick to natural, nutritional remedies when you can: They're enabling agents. Avoid drugs when you can: They're blocking agents with side effects that often fight your body's normal healing process.

In general, you'll discover your body is capable of healing itself if you give it the right stuff.

5. Get started! Check it out! Get your hands on our fascinating newsletter and put it to work.

With your subscription, you'll also get at no extra charge two rapid-results SPECIAL RE-PORTS that will kick-start your adventure in super-health:

1. *How to Have Super Energy in a World of Chronic Fatigue*

2. *21 Ways to Turn Back the Calendar (and extend your life!)*

Put the principles in these publications to work, and you'll begin to notice the effects within days. If you're like most, you'll feel more energetic than you have in years.

It doesn't take long for your anti-age fighters to kick in and get to work on rebuilding your health and even reversing any damage already done.

And after six months or so, you may begin to think you're living in someone elses body!

Get even more...

Sign up for a two-year subscription and we'll also send you two more special reports FREE:

3. *6 Alternative Treatments Your Doctor Won't Tell You About*

4. *Keeping Your Heart Young for a Century*

You'll see more about these special reports on the following pages.

And be sure to send us the enclosed reply form. You must not miss the next exciting issues of *Dr. Atkins' Health Revelations*. They will change your life for the better, enabling you to prevent many of today's serious illnesses before they strike.

And just as important, they may point out an effective treatment for some disorder you already have, one you had resigned yourself to.

You'll be reading about treatments that work. I know they work because I see patients improving every hour of every day. That's why those of us in Complementary Medicine put up with opposition from foot-dragging traditional physicians. With patients being healed by the thousands, how could we ever turn our backs on the methods that really work?

I don't want you to be surprised by suffering. Ever. And I don't want you to suddenly find yourself strapped to an operating table, waiting for the surgeons knife to descend. And I don't want you to be condemned to a life of moping around on some debilitating drug, less than half the person you used to be.

I want you to be running around and getting into all kinds of mischief for many years to come!

But how can you hope to escape the fate of most of your friends if you don't keep up with today's awesome discoveries? Send me the Charter Subscriber Certificate on the last page. Act now, before it's too late!

Yours for a long, healthy future,

Robert C. Atkins, M.D.

Robert C. Atkins, M.D.

P.S. The cost of a subscription is almost nothing compared to what you'll probably pay in pills, doctor's fees, hospital charges, and long term invalid care if you don't get your system in balance and in good condition.

I can help you. And the experts say that the government's ambitious plans will likely drive them up further. Medicare is in trouble already. Unless you are quite well off, you'll not be able to pay for even one long-term illness. Isn't it worth a few cents a day to feel like a million and stay well?

Seven Reasons to Join Our Healthy Readers Today

1. Conventional medicine is unable to stop the rise in major diseases: cancer, heart disease, diabetes, hypertension, arthritis, and more. Complementary Medicine has answers that work.

2. Health care costs are skyrocketing. You can't afford to contract a major disease, and you need good information to help you stay healthy and robust for your entire, long life.

3. The food and drug industries are economically motivated to feed you overprocessed, fat-free foods and then sell you drugs to combat the resulting disease. You need to be part of a strong movement to fight back, to resist their stranglehold on your nutritional choices.

4. You need access to a full range of current, valid health information, so you are not confused by the medical/state propaganda machine. For instance, it's a safe bet that no one has told you that many large medical studies have shown beyond a doubt that low cholesterol is a powerful precursor of cancer.

5. If you rely on most health publications, you will be subjected to opinions that are tightly controlled by major medical schools, agribusiness, giant pharmaceutical houses, or the government. Sometimes they act in your best interest, sometimes their own.

6. Some medical publications are boring and unreadable. And often unusable. You'll find *Dr. Atkins' Health Revelations* exciting and highly useful. We guarantee it.

7. Freebies!
As a subscriber, you'll receive various gifts and benefits from time to time. To start with, you'll get:

■ At least 12 monthly issues full of nutritional and medical breakthroughs with *Dr. Atkins' Health Revelations*

■ Up to 5 life-changing special reports full of health breakthroughs your doctor won't know for at least 10 more years! (Keep reading for more details.)

■ 25% off your first purchase (no matter how large) of nutritional supplements from Complementary Formulations

■ 20% off Dr. Atkins' current best seller, *Dr. Atkins' New Diet Revolution*

FREE Bonus Report #1
21 Ways to Turn Back the Clock

If you want to live a VERY long time ... if you want those years to be active, healthy, and free of pain ... if you want to be mentally alert, free from worry over osteoporosis, heart attacks, arthritis, or Alzheimer's disease ... you will want to read this special report.

It's the program I follow, and it's kept me active, healthy, and energetic enough to run a 6-floor outpatient clinic in New York ... host America's longest-running radio health program ... write 6 health and diet books ... and still have energy left over to exercise regularly and relax with my wife!

Does my program guarantee you <u>perfect</u> health? Of course not, but it will give you most everything you need to live to a happy and ripe old age. I intend to do just that, and it gives me pleasure to imagine you marching alongside me, achieving the same results.

For instance, I'll show you how to help ... keep your mind alert, and your memory as sharp as a tack ... for decades to come!

A few years ago, a nutritionally-based medicine was introduced as a treatment for senility, and I believe this super nutrient could turn out to be one of the greatest breakthroughs in brain medicine!

Long-term studies have shown this safe, no-side-effect substance—taken from a fungus that grows naturally on rye and other grains—helps to provide **significant improvement in memory and learning ability**. Over 22 studies have shown that, astonishingly, this substance can aid in ...

- Improving oxygen supply to the brain
- Improving brain metabolism
- Protecting brain cells from free radical damage
- Slowing the deposit of age pigment in the brain

I'll tell you all about this breakthrough substance—including how much can help you maintain your alert and active mind for decades to come in *21 Ways to Turn Back the Clock*.

I'll also tell you about ...

Three super nutrients that nourish your NEW and improved body

I've been taking them regularly for years ... and I'm convinced that they've played a significant role in allowing me to continue enjoying a vigorous and active life. I recommend you **take them every day to rejuvenate and protect your body**.

One is an ancient trace mineral used widely in Japan as an energy booster and pain killer ... as well as a preventive for cancer. It stimulates the activity of many key immune system chemicals, such as the macrophages, lymphocytes, and interferon production.

One has been a staple of Chinese herbal medicine for thousands of years ... and, in fact, has been an important resource for many pharmacological chemicals—including some that are bactericidal, fungicidal, immune-enhancing, and even anti-allergic!

And one is an herb used widely in other cultures as a tonic: a health balancer that provides energy, combats physical and emotional stress, and even helps boost mental ability!

Plus, in this special report packed with life-lengthening secrets, you'll discover ...

- Why one of the very best life extenders is also the most enjoyable: It could help double your chances of living a long and healthy life!

- One of the most serious risk factors for ill health and a short life: How to know if you have it ... and how you CAN work to reverse it immediately!

- The **Eskimos' secret** to low heart disease rates: You don't have to move to Alaska to get the same protection!

- My most recommended vitamin and mineral program. Scientists believe humans have the potential to live a full 120 years—if it weren't for free-radical damage! This daily program is one of the most powerful and <u>comprehensive</u> way to battle free radicals ... and give you a good shot at those extra decades!

• The ancient oriental "miracle tree" herb that fights off vascular disease, depression, headaches, hearing loss and more! You can get it in your local health food store today!

FREE Bonus Report #2
How to Have Super Energy in a World of Chronic Fatigue

Right now, you can walk into any health food store and ask for this amino acid supplement that not only <u>transforms fat into energy</u> for muscular activity ... it also has side-benefits for your heart: it helps raise the levels of your heart-protective HDL cholesterol!

As a doctor who's had patients streaming through his office for thirty years, I can tell you that fatigue is a No. 1 health complaint. With so many new advances in nutritional research— and the dozens of safe, side-effect-FREE energizing nutrients out there today—you can bet the Atkins Center has found plenty of ways to reverse the most common health complaint in North America!

Fact is, your body is a superb mechanism with incredible potential for energy and activity. Given the chance, with the right nutrition and nutritional supplements ... you could transform yourself into one of those people who dashes around with the energy and drive of a typical teenager pepped up on youthful hormones and perfect health!

The nutritional advice contained in this special report ... can help you astonish everyone you know. Forget the very meaning of the word fatigue!

In this special report, I'll show you how you can reverse the most common causes of fatigue: from the **candida yeast** and **chronic infection** ... to **prescription medications** that steal your stamina and sneaky **food allergies** or **food intolerances** most doctors don't diagnose.

Then I'll take you to the next level: <u>super energy</u>.

I'll tell you about the most effective herbs, vitamins, enzymes, and amino acids that can dramatically improve energy and endurance. I'll even tell you about the **high-powered nutrient program** I recommend to my patients with chronic fatigue. These are the nutrients that help re-establish the strength and viability of your immune system ... and provide you with natural long-lasting energy!

Get Health Revelations for Two Years and Get Two More Exciting Bonus Gifts . . .

FREE Bonus Report #3
Keeping Your Heart Young
For A Century

The very thought of a heart bypass—your chest open to the air, your rib cage spread apart, your brain and body dependent upon the efficiency of a heart lung machine, and the possibility of sudden death—is a terrifying one indeed. It could easily be you on the operating table. Thousands of Canadians end up there every year.

That's why you MUST learn today how to keep your heart strong, your arteries clear, and your blood pumping powerfully throughout your body. At the Atkins Center, we produce dramatic results every day with our heart disease patients ... *without* drugs or surgery.

In this special report, you'll discover the Atkins Center's defense against heart disease ... they're simple, pain-free, and much more effective than any cholesterol drug or angioplasty balloon! For example ...

- **One of the most important nutrients for heart health**: I've seen this mineral do just about everything a heart medication can do—without any risk of adverse effects. It can help stabilize heart rhythm, prevent coronary spasm, control blood pressure, and cut down on complications after a heart attack.

- Only a few years ago, scientists pinpointed a substance that **allows artery walls to relax and expand**, helping blood to flow more easily. This substance turned out to be nitric acid (not the nitrous oxide gas you get from the dentist.) Nitric oxide is readily and exclusively derived from an amino acid we get in high-protein foods ... or in supplements. I'll tell you what that amino acid is, because not only does it relax blood vessels, it's also been shown to inhibit platelet and cell clumping in rabbits!

- You can **improve your total cholesterol ratio**, relieve **chest pain** or **exertion pain**, reverse and **prevent free radical damage** to your heart and arteries, and even **stabilize your blood sugar** levels ... I'll tell you which herbs, vitamins, minerals, essential oils, and amino acids work best for which conditions. And I'll also give you my **basic daily heart protective nutrient program**!

I'll also give you complete details on the miraculous chelation therapy. Nothing in my career has been more amazing to me than the clinical success I've had with chelation! On a case-by-case basis, 80% improve overall functioning of their heart and nearly half reverse completely their heart disease! I'll tell you all

about it, where to go to get it, and how to know
if it's right for you!

I'll also tell you about many "health foods"
that wear down your system over time—foods
that disturb your insulin levels, clog your arteries, induce mood swings and frequent illness.
For instance, even though margarine contains
no cholesterol, it still does serious damage to
your heart and arteries! The famed Harvard
Nurses Study found that eating margarine in-
creases the number of deaths from heart disease by 66 percent! I'll show you why, and then
I'll show you how to pick out the naturally rich
and flavorful fats and oils that are GOOD for
your heart.

Caution! If, after a few weeks on the nutrition plan that's right for you ... you notice your
symptoms start fading ...

- Your cholesterol comes down
- Your blood pressure stabilizes
- Your blood sugar is stabilizing
- You lose those 15 pounds ...

... do <u>NOT</u> change or go off any medication on
your own! You must work with your doctor, *especially* if you have a heart condition or are diabetic.

FREE Bonus Report #4:
Six Alternative Treatments Your
Doctor Won't Tell You About

Medical breakthroughs ... underground treatments ... "miracle panaceas" ... that's what you'll discover within the pages of this urgent special report I've prepared for all *Health Revelations* subscribers. For example ...

Did you know that there are over 100 well-founded, scientifically based cancer therapies that are safer and work <u>better</u> than mainstream therapies? For example, there's an anticancer herbal formula made of North American herbs that's been used for centuries by the Native American Cree tribe. <u>Virtually all of my cancer patients who drink this tea regularly report they feel much better after just one week</u>!

Did you know that you can safely **improve your circulation** and **detoxify your entire system** with certain "oxygen-liberating" therapies that Europeans have been using for over 50 years? Some studies report this health-enhancing therapy can even help control chronic illnesses! What are the risks? A recent study of 384,775 patients showed that the rate of side effects was an astonishingly low 0.0007 percent!

Did you know that it's now possible to **avoid prostate surgery** altogether ... when nutritional therapy does NOT help? This painless, inexpensive therapy is the biggest breakthrough in prostate care to come down the pike in the last several decades! The Atkins Center was one of the first medical centers in America—and remains one of the FEW— to use it!

I've been using these little-known but well-founded alternative treatments for decades. I know they're safe, and I know they work!

Medicine never stops changing. A few months from now, some of the good information you've just learned in this book will be out of date! Protect yourself for years to come by following *Dr. Atkins' Health Revelations*. Fill out the enclosed charter subscription certificate mail it in the enclosed reply envelope.

FAST REPLY BONUS FOR ALL SUBSCRIBERS!

The Secrets of the Atkins Center

This is it folks! I'm opening up the doors and letting you in on three decades of powerful health and healing secrets in use at the Atkins Center. The following list represents just a fraction of what you'll learn in this exciting new report!

- Our most important recommendation for **daily heart protection**: This vitamin alone can help protect your heart for decades. In a recent Harvard study, those who took this vitamin enjoyed a decrease in their heart disease rates that was six times greater than the most effective results ever achieved with a traditional cholesterol-lowering program!

- Attention women: I'll give you the KEY to overcoming your **menopause** symptoms *without* increasing your breast cancer risk. If you're already taking estrogen, I'll show you how to minimize, possibly completely eliminate your estrogen dosage ... simply by adding two safe hormone-balancing nutritional supplements.

- If you suffer with **arthritis**, I'll show you six steps you can take to alleviate your pain ... and nine supplements that practically <u>guarantee</u> pain-free joints and a comfortable, easy range of motion.

- The 7-second secret to drug-free **headache relief**: Use this quick, easy-to-learn technique to release endorphins into your bloodstream that can relieve your headache.

- The remarkable nutrient that combats **varicose veins** *and* **allergies**! This natural substance derived from pine tree bark is a great antioxidant, too!

- The Atkins Center "trick" to putting an end to **after-dinner snack binges**. This time-tested proven solution can also get rid of your sweet tooth, to boot!

- **WARNING!** Some blood pressure drugs are harmful to your memory! If you're taking medication for high blood pressure, there are two very popular drugs that have recently been shown to <u>impair verbal memory</u> in both normal and hypertensive patients! I'll tell you what they are ... and I'll also show you how you can lower your blood pressure <u>without</u> medication found to date.

- Plus, our non-surgical solutions to prostate enlargement, Crohn's disease, colitis, clogged arteries, and more!

Send in your reply coupon within the next ten days, and I'll rush you this special report FREE!

No-Risk Introductory Subscription Offer
(For new subscribers only)

☐ **BEST DEAL!** Rush all four FREE reports, including *Keeping Your Heart Young for a Century* and *6 Alternative Treatments Your Doctor Won't Tell You About*, and enter my two-year trial subscription (24 issues) to *Dr. Atkins' Health Revelations* for $89 (regularly $154). (See reverse for more about FREE reports.) I'm also entitled to 20% off Dr. Atkins' current best seller, *Dr. Atkins' New Diet Revolution.*

☐ **GREAT DEAL:** I prefer a one-year subscription to *Dr. Atkins' Health Revelations* for $59 (regularly $104). Please rush me my two free reports, *21 Ways to Turn Back the Calendar* and *How to Have Super Energy in a World of Chronic Fatigue.* My one-year trial subscription also entitles me to 20% off Dr. Atkins' current best seller, *Dr. Atkins' New Diet Revolution.*

☐ **Quick-Reply Bonus Gift!** I'm replying within 10 days. Please send me *The Secrets of the Atkins Center.*

Return your order to: *Health Revelations* • P.O. Box 1051 • Fort Erie, ON L2A 5N8
(410) 783-8440 • Fax (410) 783-8438

☐ My payment for $59($89 for two years) is enclosed. (Make checks payable to Health Revelations. 7% GST included.)

☐ Charge my credit card: ☐VISA ☐MasterCard ☐AMEX

Card #: _____

Expiration Date: _____

Signature: _____

Name: _____

Address: _____

City/Province/Postal Code _____

Telephone: _____
(In case we have a question about your order.)

FREE WITH YOUR ONE-YEAR SUBSCRIPTION

21 Ways to Turn Back the Calendar:

Dr. Atkins' personal program for rejuvenation, based on 40 years of successful experiences. He will tell how to avoid the scourges of later life—osteoporosis, arthritis, and Alzheimer's disease, an easy nutritional program...with a 90% success rate, how to cut the likelihood of death from heart disease, and more.

How to Have Super Energy in a World of Chronic Fatigue:

Dr. Atkins will walk you step by step through the four reasons people experience fatigue, and then shows you how to transform your lethargy into the kind of zing you once had.

You'll also receive 20% OFF a copy of Dr. Atkins' latest best seller, *Dr. Atkins' New Diet Revolution.*

FREE WITH YOUR 2-YEAR SUBSCRIPTION

Keeping Your Heart Young for a Century:

You'll see first hand the latest secrets that science is uncovering and how Dr. Atkins uses them at the Atkins Center for Complementary Medicine.

Six Alternative Treatments Your Doctor Won't Tell You About:

Dr. Atkins outlines some of the greatest lessons we've learned which you can put into practice immediately...to help treat the "untreatable."

For fastest service, please fax your order to: [1-410] 783-8438

No-Risk Introductory Subscription Offer
(For new subscribers only)

☐ **BEST DEAL!** Rush all four FREE reports, including *Keeping Your Heart Young for a Century* and *6 Alternative Treatments Your Doctor Won't Tell You About*, and enter my two-year trial subscription (24 issues) to *Dr. Atkins' Health Revelations* for $89 (regularly $154). (See reverse for more about FREE reports.) I'm also entitled to 20% off Dr. Atkins' current best seller, *Dr. Atkins' New Diet Revolution*.

☐ **GREAT DEAL:** I prefer a one-year subscription to *Dr. Atkins' Health Revelations* for $59 (regularly $104). Please rush me my two free reports, *21 Ways to Turn Back the Calendar* and *How to Have Super Energy in a World of Chronic Fatigue*. My one-year trial subscription also entitles me to 20% off Dr. Atkins' current best seller, *Dr. Atkins' New Diet Revolution*.

☐ **Quick-Reply Bonus Gift!** I'm replying within 10 days. Please send me *The Secrets of the Atkins Center*.

☐ My payment for $59($89 for two years) is enclosed. (Make checks payable to Health Revelations. 7% GST included.)

☐ Charge my credit card: ☐VISA ☐MasterCard ☐AMEX

Card #: _____

Expiration Date: _____

Signature: _____

Name: _____

Address: _____

City/Province/Postal Code _____

Telephone: _____
(In case we have a question about your order.)

Return your order to: *Health Revelations* • P.O. Box 1051 • Fort Erie, ON L2A 5N8
(410) 783-8440 • Fax (410) 783-8438

FREE WITH YOUR ONE-YEAR SUBSCRIPTION

21 Ways to Turn Back the Calendar:

Dr. Atkins' personal program for rejuvenation, based on 40 years of successful experiences. He will tell how to avoid the scourges of later life—osteoporosis, arthritis, and Alzheimer's disease, an easy nutritional program...with a 90% success rate, how to cut the likelihood of death from heart disease, and more.

How to Have Super Energy in a World of Chronic Fatigue:

Dr. Atkins will walk you step by step through the four reasons people experience fatigue, and then shows you how to transform your lethargy into the kind of zing you once had.

You'll also receive 20% OFF a copy of Dr. Atkins' latest best seller, *Dr. Atkins' New Diet Revolution.*

FREE WITH YOUR 2-YEAR SUBSCRIPTION

Keeping Your Heart Young for a Century:

You'll see first hand the latest secrets that science is uncovering and how Dr. Atkins uses them at the Atkins Center for Complementary Medicine.

Six Alternative Treatments Your Doctor Won't Tell You About:

Dr. Atkins outlines some of the greatest lessons we've learned which you can put into practice immediately...to help treat the "untreatable."

100% Anytime Money-Back Guarantee

Long term, you will save far more in medical expenses than you'll ever pay in subscription fees. If you ever feel the newsletter is not living up to this promise, you will get a full pro-rated refund on all unmailed issues. No problems, no hassles, no questions.

For fastest service, please fax your order to: [1-410] 783-8438